Fibroid Tumors Healed Naturally

A Personal Journey Shared
With
Specific How-To's

Faye Hardaway

PositiveWay, In   Atlanta, Georgia

FIBROID TUMORS HEALED NATURALLY

A Personal Journey Shared With Specific How-To's

by Faye Hardaway

Let us hear from you. If you find the information in this book to be helpful, please write us at the address below. Thank you

Published by:

PositiveWay, Inc.
Post Office Box 310115
Atlanta, Georgia 31131-0115
USA

orders: PosWayInc@aol.com
(404) 691-5107   fax (404) 691-7119

Library of Congress Control Number: 2004092318

ISBN: 0-9662663-7-4

First Printing 2004

Printed in the United States of America

Dedication

This book is dedicated to *all* the *women (our ancestors, present warriors and future generations)* who have experienced/endured the uterine fibroid tumor challenge.

My prayer is that women be healed of any and all challenges with their menses.

Thank God
from whom
all blessings
flow

Acknowledgments

All women of the world, and the men who love them (my father, Hulit Hardaway, being one of the greatest). With a special thanks to my mother, Joyce Hardaway, grandmother, Rosa Ellis, late grandmother, Lottie Hardaway, aunts Connie Martin, Christine Pace and Virginia Ellis (who gave much assistant), sisters Sheral Hardaway-Kemp-Mizell (proofreader), Betty Banks, Angelique Griggs and Janice McKinney, my goddaughters Angela, Kimyanna, Candice and Jasmine, Jeanette Sheppard (proofreader), Tazar Gissentanner, Cassandra Wells, Ph.D., Rev. Sylvia Hall, Adrienne Sabir-Hudson and all other family, friends and well-wishers who provided encouragement through kind words and/or other deeds as I worked on this book.

Anthony Timmons, Sketches
Phyllis Mueller, Copy Editor (front and back cover)
Ithan Payne and Duey Pham, Cover Design

May many blessings flow back to you.

Foreword

The Technological Revolution has given us great advances in technology and improved our overall standard of living. However, these same advances have caused us to rely on modern science, technology and medicine to cure all of our illnesses and reverse the consequences of years of poor diet and lifestyle choices.

Focusing on technological advances in medicine has defocused our attention on the body's amazing ability to heal and restore itself if given the appropriate building blocks. Faye Hardaway discovers the amazing power of the body through a sometimes agonizing journey through the mine field of modern medicine. Ms. Hardaway's journey takes her on a journey where she visits seventeen doctors some suggesting that she have a hysterectomy. Ms. Hardaway's faith, determination and perseverance allowed her to continue believing that her body could heal itself if she did everything she could, physically and spiritually to promote the process. Ms. Hardaway is the modern day "woman with the issue of blood." The woman in this New Testament story had visited several doctors, spent all her money but was worse not better. She fought through the crowd and touched the hem of Jesus' garment and was healed. Jesus said that her faith healed her. Ms. Hardaway's faith and determination have also healed her.

Eldred B. Taylor, M.D.
Author of
Are Your Hormones Making You Sick?

Warning—Disclaimer

Table of Contents

As your faith is strengthen you will find that there is no longer the need to have a sense of control, that things will flow as they will, and that you will flow with them, to your great delight and benefit.

—Emmanuel—

1

HOW I DISCOVERED I HAD UTERINE FIBROID TUMORS

It had been a typical hectic workday. As I drove home around 6:30 p.m. (a little earlier for me than the time I normally left the office) and started approaching the downtown area of Atlanta, Georgia, a talk show was on the radio. I was not really focusing on the talk show, I was just happy to be off early, thrilled that there was no rush hour traffic and was admiring the buildings. The talk show was one of those health type shows and I overheard the gentlemen who was the guest saying white flour and a list of other things were not good for you. He then went on to list the symptoms of uterine fibroid tumors. He said, "Heavy periods, clots, lasting for seven days." I said, aloud in the car, "I have that...those symptoms. I better call a doctor tomorrow and check this out."

That was my beginning into the world of uterine fibroid tumors. And, it was a twelve (12) year journey for me.

I had always been a healthy eater. I was in my early thirties (this point becomes important later as you learn more about this dis-ease), I had never been married, never had children and was very close to becoming a vegetarian. I exercised daily. In fact, I had been an aerobics instructor and a personal trainer. My mother laughs as she often tells the story of me running around the backyard every evening when I was in high school long before running—jogging as it later was fashionably called—became popular.

As you can see, I was one who cared about my body. Up until this point, I rarely went to the doctor, not even for annual checkups. I didn't need to. I was healthy. I have always been one to believe in natural ways. More doctors (referring to American doctors) are becoming in-tuned with preventive care than they have been in the past. This is a good move.

On the following morning of hearing the talk show, I pulled out a telephone book to find a doctor—a gynecologist. My selection criteria, it would have to be a woman....someone who would understand. So, with a few other particulars, I made a selection. I called the doctor's (a woman) office and the receptionist answered. I told her about what I had heard on the radio and told her what my periods were like (heavy flow, lasting for seven days). The receptionist very cheerfully and nonchalantly said, "Oh, you have fibroids and are going to have to have a hysterectomy." Wow! What a way to find out.

Now, I did not know much about hysterectomies at the time, but I had heard of them and knew it was something I did not want now (I was approximately 32/33 years old) and maybe never.

I had never had any problems with my periods before. I was a late bloomer, started wearing a bra around 13 (not like some of the other girls starting at 9 years old) and my periods started when I was around 14 years old. All through my teens and twenties my periods were smooth sailing. That is one way of knowing you have fibroids, as I told one of my doctors, "In my teens and twenties I never even thought of my periods. Sure, I didn't like them, who does? However, they came on and went off without me having to make many adjustments. With fibroids, different story, *my periods began to consume too much of my life.*"

After speaking with the receptionist at the doctor's office, although I should have ran fast the other way, considering she had already told me the theme of that office—hysterectomy, I made an appointment with the doctor (a woman) anyway.

When I went to the doctor's office, I was greeted with a big smile by a lady I knew from work who was leaving the same office after an appointment. She told me that she loved the doctor, "She (the doctor) gave me my hysterectomy," the lady said.

The doctor came into the room where I was undressed and already positioned on the table for what I felt would be a routine office exam. She quickly inserted her fingers into my vagina, pulled them out and said get dressed and come into my office for a consultation.

When I went into her office, she had removed her white doctor's jacket and was wearing regular plain clothes, which I thought was a nice idea because it seemed to have removed some of the barriers. She proceeded to tell me that I had a fibroid the size of a pea (I later found out that they usually come in clusters, like grapes...if there is one, there is usually another or others). She went on to tell me dutifully that most women have them, including herself, and that, "You will have to have a hysterectomy." She said that she has to have a hysterectomy, too, and will do it someday when she gets the time. This was the attitude I also heard later expressed through another woman—a management professional—who was a co-worker of mine. It is o.k. if you feel this way, but there are women who do not see a hysterectomy as an option for them, yet they don't know what their options are.

The purpose of this book, is to share with other women what one woman actually experienced as she searched for answers/options. But, most importantly, each woman will be left with her own personal decision to choose what is best for her.

This is not a book to persuade you one way or the other. The information as it is known to the author and personally experienced in many instances, is presented. You decide for yourself after reading it.

We used to have the art of sitting on the front porch and combing each others' hair, shelling beans or whatever else occupied our hands as we shared our experiences and remedies. Since we (women) have gone into the workplace, established professional careers and are many times the sole caregivers of children, our worlds have grown to be so fast-paced that we have forgotten to make time to talk with our friends.

Reacquaint yourself with your girlfriends, that may be the first step to your healing. Women learn from other women. Not only do we have our own innate wisdom, we are caregivers, nurturing and very supportive of each other.

I personally joined a support group with women having the same challenge. Though you may choose not to join a support group at this time, let this book become your support.

My greatest aspiration in writing this book is that readers (including you) will not have to endure the suffering and aggravation I experienced the twelve years I had the challenge of uterine fibroid tumors. You have heard of the story in the Bible of the woman with the issue of blood. I felt I was that woman. I can certainty relate to the experience.

Let me become your support group. As you read the pages, know that the author is not someone who is just presenting information, but someone who has experienced the journey and can relate to what you may be experiencing.   Peace

To get up each morning with the resolve to be happy...is to set our own conditions to the events of each day. To do this is to condition circumstances instead of being conditioned by them.

—Ralph Waldo Trine—

2

HOW DO YOU KNOW IF YOU HAVE UTERINE FIBROID TUMORS

Symptoms

- Heavy menstrual flow
- Large clots
- Long lasting periods (7 days or more)
- Spotting in-between periods
- Some women report painful intercourse, with spotting to follow
- Periods consuming too much of your life

:Note:
These are the general signs of uterine fibroid tumors. This list is not a diagnose. There may be other signs or other medical conditions requiring medical attention. See your doctor.

> *Uterine fibroid tumors are believed to be associated with estrogen...they tend to go away when a woman goes through menopause (estrogen production is over). The focus of this book is to share a unique way to decrease the amount of circulating excess estrogen when the issue is uterine fibroid tumors.*

Sometimes a woman can have uterine fibroid tumors and not know it, i. e. have no symptoms (*asymptomatic*). In this case, it might be found out via a routine examination by her doctor.

If a woman is told she has a uterine fibroid tumor and she is not having any symptoms/discomfort, there is no need to panic, but is a good indication she needs to clean up her diet.

Also, I point out here that any and all abnormal bleeding should be checked out by a doctor. Be wise.

Definitions

Uterus—the place which *holds the baby* during *pregnancy* inside a woman—sometimes called a woman's *womb*. The uterus is usually described as *"pear shaped"* (upside down). And, weighs about 6 ounces under normal circumstances.

Uterine Fibroid Tumor—a *tumor* (growth, *usually benign* (non-cancerous) located in or around the *uterus,* made of *smooth muscle tissue* and *fibrous* (stringy, ropy, gelatin like—sticky, gummy, gluey) *connective tissue.*

The texture of uterine fibroid tumors is sometimes described as *firm* or *solid.*

Other Names: uterine myomas, fibromas, leio-myomas, uterine fibroids. Common names: fibroid(s), fibroid tumor(s), "female problems."

Throughout this book the author will usually use the term "uterine fibroid tumor."

Uterine fibroid tumors, stimulated by reproductive hormones, are most likely to grow during the child-bearing/reproductive stages of a woman. With this in mind, they are known to *grow fast during pregnancy* (a time in which the body produces even more estrogen).

Locations: Uterine fibroid tumors grow in the following locations and are classified by such locations.

•Submucosal
Grow *inside* the womb
(the ones that *cause a lot* of the *excessive* bleeding challenges with uterine fibroids)

•Pedunculated
Attach to the uterus by *a stem*

•Intramural
Grow in the *uterus wall muscles*

•Suberosal neoplasms
Sprout on the *outside* of the wall of the uterus

Sizes: Uterine fibroid tumors have different sizes, and are usually referred to in terms of sizes of food, especially fruits and vegetables, like the size of a *pea, orange, grapefruit, cluster of grapes;* or objects, like a golf ball.

17

One lady shared with me that she was told she had a fibroid the size of an egg. She had lived on a farm before and looking back over this now, 43 years later, she jokingly, yet inquisitively said, "Now, I don't know what that really meant. You have different sizes of eggs, small, medium, large and extra large."

My grandmother told me of a person who once lived with her (my grandmother cared for a lot of people) who had a uterine fibroid tumor the size of a 9 lb. baby. The lady looked as though she was nine months pregnant. My grandmother said the children during that time (the 1920's) used to say the lady was that way because she had never had a child and that was her baby. She wore a homemade corset (girdle type ladies' undergarment) to try to keep it in place. The lady was in her fifties when she had the fibroid removed. An article was written about her in the small town newspaper for having the largest tumor of that time.

Some Interesting Statistics on Uterine Fibroid Tumors

- fibroids affect between 70%-80% of women

- fibroids occur in 1 out of every 4 to 5 women over the age of 35, however, women in their twenties (and younger, although not as common) can also develop them

- the reason is not yet known, but more black than white women get fibroids, for example *one study* revealed that 72% of African Americans researched had fibroids compared to 50% Caucasian women researched. Still, the numbers are alarming for both, and both have been impacted by a tradition of hysterectomies to eradicate the problem.

- fibroids are more often developed between the ages of 35 and 45

> Being overweight (eating the wrong food) increases your chances of having fibroids.

These statistics are as of the original writing of this book. It is my hope that the numbers will get better over time. They will act as a reminder. This author feels that one woman challenged with uterine fibroid tumors is one too many. You would too, if you were that woman. Let's learn together, use our wisdom and grow beyond this dis-ease.

Note: Previous statistics reflected for U.S. women. Worldwide activity would increase this epidemic significantly. Sources: Women Magazine; National Institutes of Health—National Institute of Child Health and Human Development; the National Institute of Environmental Health Sciences (NIEHS) and the National Center for Research on Minority Health and Health Disparities (NCMHD); University of Maryland Medicine; the National Uterine Fibroids Foundation; Ebony magazine; Nutrition Health Review: The Consumer's Medical Journal; The Medical Center online; MayoClinic.com and; MEDLINEplus. See references at the end of this book for more details.

Affects of Uterine Fibroid Tumors

Some women complain of *constipation* and/or *frequent urination* as a result of the locations of some fibroids, i. e. they may be pressing up against the colon and/or kidneys.

It is important for a woman with uterine fibroid tumors to address challenges with constipation because improperly eliminating causes estrogen to re-circulate in the body. Also, constipation can lead to *hemorrhoids* due to excessive straining during bowel movements.

Ways to address constipation are discussed later in this book.

However, most importantly, a woman challenged with *excessive bleeding* due to uterine fibroid tumors should have her *iron checked* periodically to ensure her iron does not get dangerously low.

Other Factors to Consider

This book addresses uterine fibroid tumors specifically, non-life threatening generally. Other factors, like life threatening diseases such as cancer may require more extreme/invasive approaches, like a hysterectomy to save the woman's life. Each woman, working with a doctor who is understanding and she can trust, must decide what is best in her specific case.

It is also pointed out here that when a woman goes in for a myomectomy, for example, she is given (<u>I was given the form right before surgery</u>) a release to sign stating, in essence, if something should go wrong (example: the person bleeds too much during the surgery) and the doctor deems it necessary, a hysterectomy may be performed. Wow, what a tough spot to be in. You are all prepped, have given your own blood, needles are stuck in you— you are ready for the surgery and this type of paper is given to you to sign. I am sure some doctors are more considerate of the timing than this.

> *Something to think about, another reason to go natural*

Today a new sun rises for me; everything lives, everything is animated, everything seems to speak to me of my passion, everything invites me to cherish it.

—Anne De Lenclos—

Sketch of a Uterus

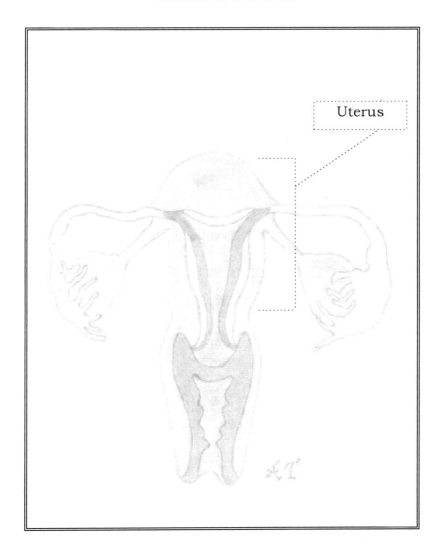

Uterus

Sketch of a Uterus With Uterine Fibroid Tumors

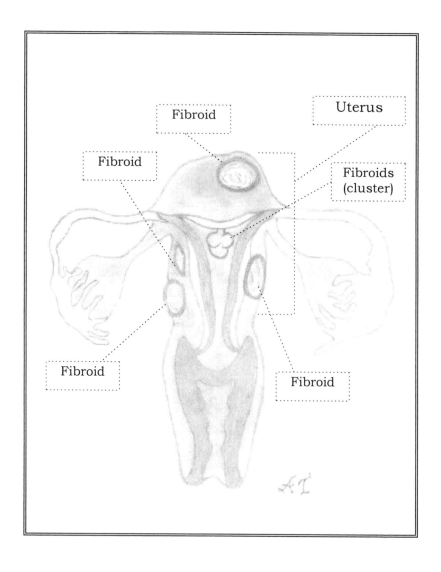

Please be advised, following are photos that may be considered graphic in nature—they reflect actual pictures of fibroid tumors which have been removed during surgical procedures.

Let seeing the pictures be an incentive to take more responsibility for the parts that we can change, like dietary factors, to help ourselves. This is not to place blame, knowingly we would not do anything to harm ourselves. Right?

Women have a lot of pride. If a woman sees a bump (pimple) on her face, she usually will do something to take care of that bump. A fibroid can be viewed as a bump (although not the same bump or lump as a pimple). Perhaps because fibroids are generally unseen, tucked away in a woman's body (although sometimes causing a woman's stomach to protrude), they have not received the healing nurturing attention that a bump on the face would have received from the same woman, but knowledge and awareness can change all of this for the better.

Think of fibroids as trapped waste/excess, they keep growing and growing because something inorganic or out of balance (in excess) can't get out.

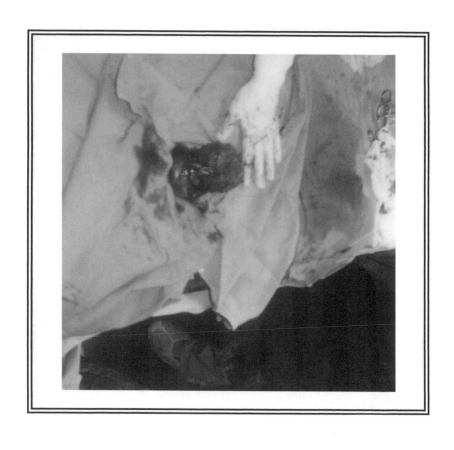

Photo Printed by Permission of the Patient

Surgery in process, large fibroid being removed. Young woman, approx. 30 years of age.

Fibroid Tumors

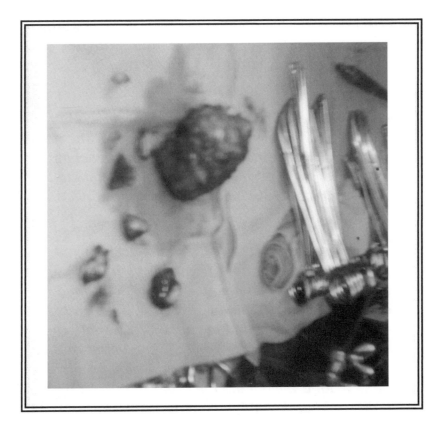

Photo Printed by Permission

This photo shows multiple fibroids that were removed.

I would like to thank the woman who provided these photos (previous and this page) so that other women may see them and learn. The fibroids shown were removed via a myomectomy.

God bless the medical doctors pure in heart who have worked so diligently in the past with what they were taught and may we (doctors and patients) all move forward to a brighter day.

I believe the best doctor is one who can teach his or her patients, in essence, "How to fish for themselves." That is, spend a lot more time teaching patients (women, in the case of this book) how to live a life more in balance with nature.

I love you—doctors—the caring ones and the not so caring ones. I have learned from you both. The caring ones showed compassion, were helpful and made the journey easier. The not so caring ones created situations in which I had to call upon strength and wisdom (intuition) from within to know better and go learn a better way for myself, and now for other women. What a blessing! I am grateful to be a part of such an exciting time when we are transcending such a barbaric past of having to have our center for creativity disturbed versus embracing our total selves with love and back to nature appropriately when it comes to healing.

Cut when you have to, but leave alone what can best be treated by natural elements of nature.

3

TRADITIONAL APPROACHES

This chapter is devoted to *summarizing* the *traditional alternatives* that have been made available to women.

Hysterectomy—The "Number One" surgery traditionally performed in the USA for women challenged with uterine fibroid tumors. Generations of women in America have had this type of surgery, especially in the black community.

This is not an attempt to attack traditional approaches, they have served their purposes in time, and still do for some women and for some situations.

Pro(s)

Eliminates the symptoms... heavy periods, etc.

Con(s)

Removes a woman's ability to have children.

Some reports of women losing their sexual desire.

Irritating, drying of the vagina area (painful sex).

No more hormones (no estrogen and no progesterone)...can throw a woman immediately into menopause—night sweats, etc.). This applies to certain types of hysterectomies.

Types of hysterectomies

Total hysterectomy—the surgical removal of the entire uterus, the fundus (the outer part of the uterus which is attached to the fallopian tubes) and the cervix.

Partial (subtotal or supracervical) hysterectomy—the uterus is removed, but the **cervix** is **left**.

Hysterectomy with <u>bilateral</u> *salpingo-oophorectomy*—the **removal** of **both ovaries**, the uterus and fallopian tubes. Ovaries removed prior to natural menopause causes immediate menopause after surgery.

Hysterectomy with <u>unilateral</u> *salpingo-oophorectomy*—some cases where only **one ovary** and **fallopian tube** are removed, along with the uterus.

Radical Hysterectomy—the top <u>portion of the vagina</u> is included in the removal process of the uterus and cervix along with other tissue around the pelvic and cervix area.

The Hysterectomy Process

A hysterectomy can be done through a woman's **abdomen** (stomach), through her **vagina** or **navel** area.

Hysterectomy via the abdomen

-longer stay in hospital

-incision/visible scarring

Hysterectomy via the vagina

-recovery is supposed to be quicker

-no visible external scarring

-may have a negative impact on sexual intercourse...the vagina may be shortened during the surgical procedure.

Hysterctomy via Laparoscopic

Incisions are made through the navel with an instrument called a "laparoscope" and the uterus is removed through the navel.

-longer surgery time because the uterus has to be removed in pieces/chunks.

However,

-shorter hospital stay

Other Traditional Surgical Approaches

Dilation and Curettage (D & C)— *dilation* means to make larger/*expanding* (the uterus is expanded) so that an instrument can be inserted to *scrape* (*curettage--scraping*) and suction out the lining of the uterus.

Myomectomy (abdominal)—fibroids are surgically removed from the uterus via surgical entry through the abdominal (stomach) area and the uterus is repaired.

> -the uterus remains intact with the woman

> -childbirth is still an option for the woman, but there may be the need for a cesarean, "C" section, for delivery. A C-section is a major surgery (abdominal—stomach area) performed instead of a vaginal delivery.

> -**fibroid tumors surgically removed may come back**, and they often do, requiring repeated surgery and/or leading eventually to a hysterectomy or the suggestion of it. The root cause of the problem needs to be dealt with—see chapter 4, natural healing.

> -excessive bleeding can happen during the surgery of a myomectomy requiring a hsyterectomy on the spot.

Like hysterectomies, there are different *types of myomectomies.*

Hysterscopic Myomectomy

Sometimes when a fibroid is protruding inside the uterus, hanging by a stem, a *fiber-optic scope* called a *hysteroscope* is inserted *through the vagina* (no external incision required) by a doctor, and with the appropriate attachment device the fibroid is cut/shaved away.

Laparoscopic Myomectomy

A probe with a camera attached and one with surgical attachments are inserted through small incisions made to a woman's *abdominal area* to remove fibroids seen via the camera.

Hysteroscopic endometrial ablation (using the rollerball electrode)—in this method the lining of the uterus (the part that sheds/bleeds each month) is burned away with a hot balloon like object. Some women have no more periods (bleeding) after this method has been performed, others have medium-to-slight to no results with this method. One major positive of this method is that the uterus remains intact.

Uterine Fibroid Embolization (UFE)—usually performed by specialized radiologists, blocking the blood supply/flow to a fibroid(s), causing the fibroid(s) to shrink.

Other—Traditional Methods

Birth Control Pills

Sometimes prescribed to help control the excessive bleeding associated with uterine fibroid tumors.

Advantage

Work for some women

Possible Side Effects

-weight gain

-blood clots

-headaches

    etc. (read the label)

Gonadotropin-Releasing Hormones (GnRH) Agonists

The hormone that is made by the hypothalamus (part of the brain) that causes estrogen to be produced is called gonadotropin-releasing hormone (GnRH), however, there are synthetically made hormones called *GnRH agonists* (drugs like *Lupron, Synarel, Zoladex...*) that can overshadow this regular process. *GnRH* (gonadotropin-releasing hormones) *agonists* are *suppressive, synthetic hormones* that work on the pituitary gland (controlled by the hypothalamus) to *shut down* the *ovaries.* When the ovaries are shut down estrogen levels decrease drastically, causing a woman to go into menopause abruptly. One doctor told me that some women say, *"Taking [name of drug] is like going to hell and back."*

On the *positive side, periods cease,* .i.e. no more heavy periods for the woman, and the fibroids shrink during the time the woman is taking the GnRH agonist. This approach is sometimes used to shrink the size of the fibroid tumor or tumors prior to surgery in order for future surgery to go smoothly for the doctor. Sometimes GnRH agonists has been given to women to bridge them over to menopause when fibroids are expected to shrink naturally due to hormonal changes in the woman. It is not recommended that a woman use a GnRH agonist for more than six (6) months, and fibroids grow back quickly once the woman stops taking the GnRH agonist if she does not naturally go into menopause.

Other Methods Tried to Alleviate the Symptoms
of Uterine Fibroid Tumors (continued)

Progesterone—The Other Side of the Equation

Progesterone is the hormone that is believed to be decreased or not produced each month of a woman's menstrual cycle during the time in which she is experiencing uterine fibroid tumors. This is a change from when both estrogen and progesterone were both being produced regularly (monthly) within the woman's cycle.

Where estrogen is believed to make things expand/grow, progesterone (the other side of the equation) is believed to make things contract. This is a balancing act of the female hormones.

Dr. Eldred B. Taylor (Atlanta, GA) is doing some wonderful work in this area.

Progestin

Synthetic progestin hormones (intent to replace progesterone) are sometimes prescribe to *help control excessive bleeding*. Drugs like *Provera, Aygestin...* fall into this category. They are usually taken during the last two weeks of a woman's cycle. Synthetic progestin works for some women, for others it does not. Read the labels for benefits and possible side effects.

Natural Progesterone

Products like *Angel Care, ProDerma, Fem Creme*...use naturally derived ingredients of progesterone. At the time of this writing you can buy these over the counter at some health food stores or through a distributor. These usually come in the form of rub on creams. It is believed that creams should have at least 400 mg of natural progesterone per oz of cream in order to be effective. There are companies like *Aeron* that test—have product integrity certification programs—the actual levels of ingredients in products. Some pharmacists (through a lot of research I found one such company—Belmar Pharmacy, Lakewood, CO) can make tablet compounds of natural progesterone, but you have to go through your doctor for a prescription.

Please note

When one is on natural progesterone, she needs to be monitored—under the care of a medical doctor. Your doctor can order for you to take a test to check your hormonal levels periodically. I had a *saliva test* called post-menopausal hormone, short that showed my *DHEA, Testosterone, estrogen (estrone, estradiol and estriol [the "good estrogen"]) and progesterone levels.*

Prostaglandin Inhibitors

Sometimes women are advised to take a *prostaglandin inhibitor* such as *ibuprofen,* like *Motrin* or *Advil*...in an effort to help control excessive bleeding. In this case, the *prostaglandin inhibitor* is to be taken few days before the menstrual cycle begins and throughout the heaviest days of the cycle. Ask your doctor for more specifics concerning your individual case.

Summary

It is believed that over time even more alternatives/options will be explored by the field of medicine to address uterine fibroid tumors.

I tried surgery (myomectomy); birth control pills [for seven months...made me fat]; synthetic and natural progesterone; extreme dietary changes, including fasting; prostaglandin inhibitors. NONE OF THESE WORKED FOR ME.

What worked for me was Prayer (belief that there was something better) and what I found by trial and error, a natural approach, I share with you in the next chapter (chapter 4).

Divine love always has met and always will meet every human need.

—Mary Baker Eddy—

4

THE NATURAL ALTERNATIVE

2 table-
spoons of
flaxseeds
daily

Other com-
ponents
Garlic
Olive Oil
Eat Your
Vegetables
Keep a Clean Colon
Get Plenty of Iron

Stay away from
Estrogen promoters
Add more foods
that block excess estrogen

I was blessed to experience two (2) occasions in which uterine fibroid tumors were releasing themselves from my body. I have the medical records to prove it! What I found out by trial & error is shared with you in this chapter.

Flaxseeds

Flaxseeds are an essential part of this natural healing plan. Do not go skimpy on this part. If you don't do anything else, ADD **TWO TABLESPOONS** OF **FLAXSEEDS DAILY** TO YOUR DIET.

Each of the two times uterine fibroid tumors were releasing themselves from my body, I asked myself what was I doing (differently) at the time of the releasing. Both times, the answer was I had added flaxseeds to my diet (two tablespoons daily). I tried to tell many medical doctors (emergency room physicians, surgeons and follow-up doctors) I had an answer. No one would listen. So, I now share it with you.

How to Use

First start with **organic** flaxseeds
(You can get these from most health food stores)

You can buy flaxseeds **whole**, already **milled** (ground), or in oil form (purchase *cold pressed* only when buying in oil form). I suggest going as close to nature as possible.

How to Grind Flaxseeds Yourself

Purchase a small (relatively inexpensive) coffee grinder

> **Step 1** Put whole, organically grown flaxseeds in the coffee grinder and grind

> **Step 2** Put ground flaxseeds in a regular blender and crumb the flaxseeds

Sprinkle ground/milled flaxseeds on food
(Do Not Cook the Flaxseeds)

Using Flaxseed Oil

Again, purchase *organic, cold pressed* flaxseed oil. Flaxseed oil must be refrigerated after it is opened. You want to see some of the flaxseed particles in the oil (shake well). You will sometimes see the words "high lignan" or "ultra high lignan" on the bottle. The more lignan, the better.

Lignan is a *fiber* and helps to decrease the amount of excess estrogen believed to cause uterine fibroid tumors.

Studies have shown that countries in which women have a high amount of lignans (flaxseed is an example, also, buckwheat and wheat) don't have the same problems with their periods and fibroid tumors; and their risk for colon and breast cancer is lower.

Adding Your Own Lignan

You can add your own lignan (flaxseed particles to your oil). Buy a relatively inexpensive bottle of organic cold pressed flaxseed oil and add some of the ground or milled flaxseeds you have made yourself.

Pour flaxseed oil

> over your favorite hot cereal
>
> over a baked white or sweet potato
>
> over a baked plantain
>
> or whatever creative idea you can come up with!

Variety

You can alternate using flaxseed oil and ground/milled flaxseeds. For example, you could have millet (some other similar grain or warm breakfast) with flaxseed oil (one tablespoon) instead of butter or margarine. And, for dinner you could have your other tablespoon of flaxseeds for the day in the form of ground/milled flaxseeds sprinkled over a salad along with your salad dressing.

You must experiment to find what you prefer to have your flaxseeds with. Each person's taste buds are different.

Recipe Suggestions

Flaxseed Smoothie

1 large banana

1 cup of strawberries

1 1/2 cup of water

1 tablespoon of flaxseeds

(can be ground/milled or whole)

1 tablespoon of crumbed sesame seeds (for calcium)

Wash fruit and cut tops off of strawberries. Place all ingredients in a blender and blend.

Yields: 1 serving

You may add more water or less depending upon your personal preference for thickness.

Also, instead of water you may substitute your favorite fruit juice, example pineapple or orange juice makes a nice blend.

Use different fruits to make it exciting.

How to crumb sesame seeds

Place 1 cup or more of *organic* whole *sesame seeds* in a regular kitchen blender and crumb. Place crumbed sesame seeds in a jar for storage in the refrigerator for future use. You can buy organic sesame seeds from most health food stores and some grocery stores in the health food/nutrition section.

Grounding/milling and crumbing flaxseeds and sesame seeds helps to break down the seeds to make them easier for you to digest. Do not put sesame seeds in a coffee grinder, they get moist and will stick in the grinder. Unlike flaxseeds (two step grounding/milling and crumbing process given previously), sesame seeds only have to be crumbed—they are a s⁻ .ter seed.

Ground/ Milled Flaxseeds & Cereal

1 bowl of whole grain cereal (example whole grain, organic corn flakes)

1 tablespoon of ground/ milled flaxseeds

1/2 cup of organic brown rice milk, vanilla flavor

Place dry ingredients in a bowl. Add rice milk (can occasionally alternate with soy milk). Enjoy!

Yields: 1 serving

DO NOT CONSUME COWS' MILK. COWS' MILK WILL ADD TO YOUR PROBLEM OF UTERINE FIBROID TUMORS. COWS ARE FED ESTROGEN HORMONES TO MAKE THEM GROW FASTER FOR MARKET. YOU DON'T NEED MORE ESTROGEN IF YOU ARE SUFFERING FROM UTERINE FIBROID TUMORS.

Flaxseed Trail Mix

1 cup of whole shelled almonds (no salt or oil added)

1 cup of organic raisins

1/2 cup of raw pumpkin seeds

1/2 cup of whole organic flaxseeds

In a dry container or bag add all ingredients together and shake. Eat as desired. The flaxseeds will be crunchy, chew them well. This makes a wonderful natural treat, especially for those having a craving for sweets.

As with all other recipes listed, the beauty is that you can be creative—make your own trail mix including nuts and dried fruits (like figs, dates...) you like.

Yields: 3 servings

Note: Raisins and currants are different. Currants are usually smaller in size and much sweeter than raisins. You decide what you like best.

Other Components

Garlic

Garlic is good for a variety of things. It is a *natural antibiotic*—it kills viruses, parasites, fungus and bacteria. It **fights against tumors**, decreases cholesterol and blood pressure, and aides in digestion.

Making a Garlic Solution

Take 5 garlic cloves from a bulb (the bulb is the entire unit)
Wash
Place cloves in a blender with 2 cups of water and blend
Store in a glass jar, with a screw on top
Refrigerate until ready to use

For Over-All Good General Health

Take one- to- two ounces of garlic solution, strain, add to a full glass (8 oz.) of water and drink. (one glass daily)

Garlic is loaded with Vitamins and Minerals

Vitamin A, B-complex, C, Sulfur, Manganese, Phosphorus, Zinc, Copper, Potassium, Calcium, Magnesium, Iron, Selenium, Germanium, Sodium and Amino Acids.

For Yeast Infections

Take Garlic Internally

Drink one glass daily as described in section for over-all good general health.

Vaginal Douche

Using one-to-two ounces of garlic solution, strain, add warm water to a douche bag and douche.

Many times garlic will remedy a vaginal yeast infection, eliminate itching and discharging, after just one application (douche). Nevertheless, listen to your body, if you need to take a garlic douche several more days, do so. Note: The garlic douching solution may cause a slight stinging sensation (it is killing germs), however, if the solution is too strong for you, add more water.

External Vaginal Itch

If you must go over the counter, for external vaginal itch relief rub a combination of an *antifungal cream*, like Lotrimin, and 1% hydrocortisone cream on the affected area.

Friendly Bacteria

Eat Yogurt (there is now *soy yogurt*) or take *acidophilus* capsules. Acidophilus (found in yogurt also) has what is called "friendly bacteria" which helps keep your digestive track clean, and you free of yeast infections. When taking acidophilus get the *non-dairy* (vegetarian) kind.

See a doctor if your problem persists to ensure there is no other problem.

Night Toddy

Take one (1) ounce of garlic solution (described previously), strain, add to a cup of water and boil for 5 minutes. Place in your favorite tea cup and drink before going to bed.

This can be your daily cup of garlic solution. Relax and have a restful night.

Eliminating Garlic Odor

If you are concerned about the possible lingering odor of garlic,

- eat a spring of parsley

- drink garlic water during a meal (preferably dinner)

- soak garlic gloves in vinegar (apple cider) and lemon solution

- squeeze lemon or lime on your tongue and swish around in your mouth

Reduce/Eliminate Saturated Fats and *Eliminate Partially Hydrogenated Fats* from Your Diet. (READ LABELS)

High fat and low fiber increases the amount of estrogen you have circulating in your system. This is not a good thing for those suffering from uterine fibroid tumors.

Monounsaturated and polyunsaturated fats are called the "good" fats because they help eliminate the "bad fats" (LDL—low density lipo proteins) which clog arteries in the body.

Olive Oil & Canola Oil

Use cold-pressed, organic olive oil or canola oil to cook with. Olive oil can be easily used in most recipes, except for when frying. Of course, deep frying is something that one should stay away from.

Olive and canola oils are both high in monounsaturated fats. Flaxseed oil is high in omega 3 fatty acids or polyunsaturated fats. Hence, the guidelines given in this program represent a balance.

Spectrum Organic Products, Inc., Petaluma, CA makes a non-hydrogenated—trans fat free, cholesterol free, relatively low in sodium, *butter-like spread* (made of canola oil, no dairy) called *Spectrum Naturals®*. Although it does not taste exactly like butter, it is a great alternative.

Much of taste preference is formed from what we are accustomed to—*habits*. Habits/actions can be modified to those more supporting of the results we desire in our lives.

Make Your Own Salad Dressing

Mix *flaxseed oil* (preferably) or olive oil with organic apple cider vinegar.

You may add your favorite herbs to taste. In various combinations, try *rosemary, thyme, garlic powder, turmeric, cumin, and cayenne pepper.* They are *good for you.*

Pour over a large green salad (green leaf lettuce, grated carrots, radish...be creative).

Sprinkle ground/milled flaxseeds and crumbed sesame seeds over and enjoy!

Stay away from sage, fennel, fenugreek, anise, or use occasionally, these herbs will promote more estrogen to circulate within your body.

Use *cayenne pepper* instead of black pepper. Cayenne pepper is healing to the stomach, black pepper is irritating.

Eat Your Vegetables

You get your daily vitamins from vegetables. Eat your vegetables. Include as many fresh vegetables as possible daily in your diet. If you can't get fresh vegetables, go with frozen. Also, eat as much raw food as possible daily—this includes fruits and vegetables.

Stay Away from Too Much Salt

Salt makes the body retain excess water—adds to bloating and makes the heart have to work harder to make the body's other organs (ex. kidneys) function properly.

Choose no-salt or low salt/low sodium (70 mg range or lower) when purchasing condiments (tomato catsup, mustard, etc.) or pre-packaged food items (such as frozen and canned goods (if you must), and snacks).

Cook as many entrees as possible with no salt. Garlic powder or granulates can be used instead of salt.

Also, a small dash of Bragg's Liquid Aminos or other salt alternatives may be added to your diet *occasionally*. Check your local health food store. Keep in mind that even if a product is relatively low in sodium, the sodium is still there so go easy on the shaker.

If you feel you must use salt occasionally, use *sea salt* when cooking only—don't add additional salt to your food. **TAKE "TABLE SALT" OFF THE TABLE.**

If you are concerned about not getting enough *iodine*, use *kelp* which is also an alternative to salt. Kelp can be kept on the table.

(note: people with hyperthyroidism or hypothyroidism may have restrictions regarding iodine. Consult your health care provider.)

Water

The type of water makes a different. You do not need to drink contaminated—germy, pesticide infested water. It is just plain unhealthy.

Use clean...*reverse osmosis* water.

Most reverse osmosis filtration (purified water) systems include carbon treatment, reverse osmosis and ultraviolet disinfection.

A sample filtration process (purified water)

Activated carbon filter—for removing chorine and odors

Micronfilter—for removing particles like dust and rust

Ultraviolet light—for disinfection

Reverse Osmosis—for removing lead, salts and other residue

Some water filtration systems repeat some of the processes, like running the water through a carbon filter a second time to help refine the taste of the water.

You can find reverse osmosis water in health food stores, and some grocery and department stores. Such stores have filtration machines, *you provide and fill your own bottles.* This is less expensive than buying the water already bottled. And, you do not have to purchase an expensive system.

Water you drink, cook or even douche with (anything you consume inside your body, especially) must be of the highest quality.

Colon Health

DRINK PLENTY OF WATER—a gallon a day. Water helps the digestive process and to soften/bring moisture to stool to help it to pass through your colon quicker. Stagnate stool/waste will cause problems...recirculation of estrogen, etc..., besides being very uncomfortable. If you have ever had the problem of constant constipation, you know what I am talking about. If you have not, count it a blessing.

> *Often women suffering from fibroid tumors also have problems with constipation, which may have been a contributing factor to the uterine fibroid tumor(s) expanding itself.*

Overcoming Constipation Naturally

Water   **Fiber**   **Oil**   **Exercise**

FIBER—There are basically three ways to get fiber naturally in your diet 1) raw fruits 2) raw vegetables (salads, juice with some added pulp, etc.) and 3) whole grains.

My Own **Natural Fiber** Recipe

2 tablespoons of wheat bran

1 large plantain

1 whole apple

1 tablespoon of flaxseeds

(ground/milled or whole)

1 tablespoon of crumbed sesame seeds

1 cup of water

Wash fruit, peel plantain, peel apple (or leave apple peel on for more added fiber), cut plantain and apple into small chunks and toss into a blender, or other type of mixer, with all other ingredients. Blend for approximately 30 seconds. Best if let stand (in the refrigerator or out) for approximately 1 hour before eating—will become creamy, gel like. Eat with a spoon and enjoy.

Yields: 1 serving

Can be eaten daily. Great as an evening treat.

The wonderful thing about the natural fiber shake is it can be eaten instead of yogurt or ice cream.

Don't forget to drink your water, especially when adding fiber to the diet.

By the way, for those having a strong craving for ice cream, try natural brands made with rice or soy, like *Rice Dream*.

CUT BACK ON NIGHTTIME EATING, especially starches. Go with fruits and vegetables in the evening. Do your best to stop eating after 10:00 p.m. Give your body time to rest and digest (process) what it has already consumed during the day. You will break the fast (breakfast) in the morning. Drink a big (8 oz.) glass of water upon rising.

Early Morning Colon Cleanser Drink

1 squeezed lime or lemon (I like lime because it has no seeds)

a pinch of cayenne pepper

1 ounce of ginger root tea

1 teaspoon of apple cider vinegar

in a tall (8 oz.) glass of warm water

Ginger Tea

2 inches of raw ginger root
3 cups of water

Wash ginger root, cut into slices, place in a blender, add water and blend (chop and liquefy). Place solution in a jar and store in refrigerator until ready to use, like in your early morning colon cleanser drink. Adding one-to-two ounces of strained ginger root tea to a cup of hot boiling water, adding 1 freshly squeezed lime or lemon, makes a lovely hot beverage. You can also drink the same solution cold (room temperature). In either case, honey may be added to sweeten (optional). Ginger root aids in overall digestion, remarkably working against gas, and is found in the produce section of most grocery stores.

WALK, WALK, AND WALK. Take a 20 to 30 minute walk daily. It helps get things *moving in the colon,* besides helping to keep you *fit, shapely, and energized.*

EAT A SALAD A DAY. Want a tremendous change for the better if challenged with constipation, EAT A SALAD A DAY....IT WILL KEEP CONSTIPATION AWAY. Green leaf lettuce as a base for better results. Flaxseed oil with ground flaxseeds sprinkled over with apple cider vinegar as a dressing.

ADD **SPROUTED WHOLE GRAIN BREAD** (low sodium or no sodium), example *Ezekiel* brand, to your diet. Great for making sandwiches.

Drinking a glass of *yellow root* tea occasionally as needed is also a good remedy for constipation, and an overall good feeling in the stomach. Yellow root twigs can be purchased from health food stores and is plentiful in the south, like Georgia, USA.

Wash a handful of yellow root twigs and place them in a pot of water, cover and boil for 20 minutes or until the water is a nice deep yellow color. Strain and pour into your favorite tea cup and sip. Store remaining yellow root tea/twigs in the refrigerator after cooling in a jar. The twigs can be used many times by adding more water to the roots in the jar while stored.

WHEN ALL ELSE FAILS, TAKE 1 TABLESPOON OF POWDERED *MAGNESIUM* (from elemental magnesium citrate), like *Natural Calm*™ brand which has 615 mg per 3 teaspoons, in a warm glass of water before going to bed or upon rising. If your bowels do not move within 24 hours repeat the process.

A Sample Diet to Overcome Chronic Constipation

Morning

> 1 bowl of cooked Millet with flaxseed oil and
> ground flaxseeds
> Apple

Mid-day/lunch

> 2 almond mixed with peanut butter, maple
> syrup sandwiches on sprouted whole grain
> bread
> Vegetable

Snack

> Apple or other piece of fruit

Evening/dinner

> Salad with flaxseed oil, ground flaxseeds & apple
> cider vinegar
> Vegetable
> Kale (or other green leafy vegetable) and carrot
> juice

Snack

> Fruit, hot natural tea (no caffeine), water or
> lemon and water

Simple, Easy Clean-Up Way to Make Homemade Vegetable Juice

1 carrot
2 leaves of green leaf vegetable (example Kale or spin-
ach)
2 leaves of green leaf lettuce
1 apple (to enhance the taste)
3 cups of water

Wash all vegetables and apple thoroughly and cut into chunks. Place in a commercial grade Vita Mixer (brand name by Vita-Mix Corporation, Olmsted Falls, Ohio) or your favorite home blender, add water, cover and place on low speed, medium speed and high speed for approx. a minute totally. Turn off mixer/blender and pour mixture through a strainer into a glass. Mash mixture in strainer with a larger spoon. Some of the small particles of the pulp from the juice should be in the juice. Drink and enjoy.

Yields: 1 Serving

This method is easier, especially clean up, than using a juicer and requires fewer ingredients (less costly). For example, it could take as many as six (6) carrots to get one glass of juice using a juicer (juice extractor) versus one (1) carrot using the method previously described (mixer/blender) and you are getting added fiber, too.

Note: *Only add apples to vegetable juices.* Other fruits will interfere with the digestive process if added to vegetable juice.

For a nice pick-me-up after a long day, add celery (1 stalk) to your juice.

Make Drinking Water Fun

- Add a little squeezed lemon (lemon twist)
- Get a beautiful water bottle, keep it in your car or take it wherever you go

---

Note: Water should be consumed at room temperature, drinking cold water shocks the body.

Iron

Getting enough iron is a must if you are experiencing heavy bleeding during your cycles. Look for natural ways to get your iron.

Daily

Eat a hefty portion of dark green, leafy vegetables (collards, kale, turnip greens, etc.) with your lunch and dinner

Put a green vegetable (spinach, etc.) in your homemade vegetable juice

Eat a salad (raw) with a dark green, leafy vegetable added

On days of your cycle, and a few days afterwards

Add *more* dark green, leafy vegetables (may be in the form of juice for quick absorption)

and/or

Add *wheat grass* juice to your diet

The thing that green plants have in common is *chlorophyll*, along with essential fatty acids, calcium, magnesium, vitamin C, manganese, vitamin A, iron, potassium and proteins. With chlorophyll, green plants absorb sunlight and transform it into energy.

The make up of chlorophyll is similar to that of human blood—hemoglobin, differing in only one molecule at the center.

Hemoglobin (Carbon, Hydrogen, Oxygen, Nitrogen and I*ron* as the *center*)

Chlorophyll (Carbon, Hydrogen, Oxygen, Nitrogen and *Magnesium* as the *center*)

Chlorophyll reduces tumors and anemia.

> *When feeling tired and sluggish, eat something green.*

Dr. Ann Wigmore, Living Foods Lifestyle™ founder and director, called chlorophyll the "blood of the plant."

Wheatgrass is a source of chlorophyll and is loaded with digestive enzymes.

My Own Process for Making Wheatgrass Juice

1 handful of organically grown wheatgrass
2 cups of water

Wash wheatgrass, cut into 1 inch sections, place in a Vita-Mixer™, add water and mix using three different speeds (low, medium and high) for approximately 2 minutes total. Strain juice, squeezing the remaining fiber with your hand into a cup, and drink.

Yields: 2 servings

When asking around, I was told you can only press the juice out of wheatgrass using a wheatgrass presser. Again, I found myself in the kitchen using my own God given imagination and creativity (you have the same) to find a better way. I found the aforementioned way to be simpler, therefore, I do it more often.

To find out more about wheatgrass, read *The Wheatgrass Book* by Dr. Ann Wigmore.

When Trying to Build Your Blood

Take two tablespoons of unsulfured *blackstrap molasses* daily in a class of water. I have known people to do this when preparing to give blood for surgery. It works! Of course, by faith and adjusting your diet and lifestyle you will not need surgery, but you still can use blackstrap molasses daily to help you with iron. I don't prefer this method because it adds a lot of sugar (although natural) to your diet.

Nursing mothers preferring a natural approach to ensure they get enough iron also benefit from adding blackstrap molasses to their diet. Blackstrap molasses is likewise used in making natural formulas for babies.

Comfortable, loose fitting clothes

Wear comfortable, loose fitting clothes, especially on days of your cycle. Your clothes do make you—they make you comfortable or miserable.

Wearing loose fitting clothing does not mean unattractiveness. Brands, like Chico's® are loose, comfortable, professional and stylist. They even have a collection that will not wrinkle when you travel. Throw on a hat, with an attitude, and you have class!

> Wearing comfortable, loose fitting clothing gives you a sense of freedom, freedom to be uniquely you, expressive and creative.

> *For Reducing Bloating/ Water Retention*
>
> *1 tablespoon of* **apple cider vinegar** *in a glass of water helps reduce bloating/water retention during menses.*

100% Cotton

Go with 100 % cotton (especially for underwear—panties and bras, including the stitching) or other natural fabrics.

Natural Remedy for Bladder Infections

*Boil 2 cups of **whole cranberries** in 6 cups of water for 20 minutes, or until cranberries pop and water turns berry red. Let cool, strain (mashing cranberries) and drink. Makes 6 servings, serving size 1 cup.* Do not substitute for preprocessed cranberry juice that is mixed with artificial flavors, sugars and preservatives. Whole cranberries can be purchased when in season and frozen for later use. Honey can be added to the recipe as a sweetener.

Flat Shoes

Flat/low heel shoes are just better for you, especially when your cycle is on. High heel shoes will make you flow/blood gush out more, creating discomfort and the fear of an embarrassing accident/spill-over happening.

No heavy lifting on days of your cycle. Heavy lifting will cause heavy bleeding.

Every day is a good day to pamper yourself, especially when your cycle is on.

Natural Fragrances, Lotions, Deodorants and Makeup

Wear natural fragrances, lotions, deodorants and makeup.

> What you put on your skin goes through your pores into your blood stream!

Fragrances

Use natural scented oils, with no alcohol. Alcohol dries the skin of its natural oils. There are cases when alcohol may be needed, this is not one of those cases.

Natural scented oils can be purchased from health food stores and some quaint specialty shops. Shop around, go on the internet. Check out the ingredients and go from there. *Auric Blends* has a nice Fine Perfume Oils line. There are others.

Let the adventurous part of you come out, experiment with mixing different fragrances, adding olive oil to tone down/dilute as needed.

Lotions

Make your own lotion/all purpose body oil by adding a little (1/2 teaspoon or more or less based upon your preference for a stronger or lighter all purpose body oil) natural scented fragrance oil to 1 & 1/2 cup of organic, cold pressed olive oil. Place in a beautiful container, cover and call it your natural all purpose body oil.

Deodorants

Use natural deodorant. Many are made with natural mineral salts, come in crystal type sticks (preferably), sprays, like *Crystal*.™ *Alba* by Alba Botanica® has a solid, organic, hypo-allergenic deodorant.

Do not use antiperspirants. They clog your sweat glands, keeping you from sweating which is a natural part of you. Sweating is another way the body cleanses/releases itself of impurities.

Anti-Acne

Mix one part Witch Hazel with one part Hydrogen Peroxide, shake
Store in container until ready for usage

Wash face with cloth and water only. Pour anti-acne solution (about the size of a quarter) on the corner of a wet face cloth and pat on face. Apply all purpose olive body oil (you make) to face and go.

Make-up

You will find that when you have cleaned up your diet (eating more naturally), adding fresh vegetable juice (with carrot as a base) daily, drinking plenty of water (at least 6-8, 8 oz. glasses a day or more), applying anti-acne solution and natural olive oil to your face after washing, you will not need as much make-up, if any at all. You will glow with natural beauty. Add some *natural lipstick* and/or *eye color* if desired. If you feel you must use a foundation, go with a foundation with natural ingredients or at least water base.

If you have been or are challenged with uterine fibroid tumors, whatever is on the list of *estrogen promoters* to *avoid* taking *internally*, do the same *externally*.

Read Labels

Stay Away from	Add more
Estrogen Promoters/	Estrogen Blockers/
Pro-Estrogenic	Anti-Estrogenic

Licorice	*Fruits (including citrus)*
Dong Quai	*Vegetables*
Sage	***Flaxseed***
Fenugreek	*Whole wheat*
Red Clover	*Buckwheat*
Ginseng	*Wheat bran* *(but not wheat germ)*
Wild Yam	
Primrose oil	
Anise	
Black Cohosh	
Fennel	
Suma	
Cow's milk *(sometimes called whey)*	
Boron	

FIBER, FIBER, FIBER
Helps rid the body of
excess estrogen

Lignins---anti-
estrogenic
Along with flaxseeds,
whole grains and bran,
cabbage, peaches, pears,
strawberries, legumes
(dried beans & peas) are
also sources of lignins.

Phyllis A. Balch, C. N. C. and James F. Balch, M. D.'s book *Rx Prescription for Cooking & Dietary Wellness*, Revised (1992), among other sources, was very instrumental in helping me identify many of the estrogen blockers, especially, and promoters. I recommend reading this book to anyone looking for a general overall healthy way of eating.

Wheat germ, although a good source of vitamin E, will make your cycles noticeably heavier. Avoid.

Also, be aware that *pesticides* contain properties that mimic estrogen, adding to excessive levels of estrogen.

Stay away from things (previous list provided) that support and pro-mote the creation of excess estrogen in your body, and add more things that help to de-crease the amount of estrogen circu-lating in your body, if you have been or are currently chal-lenged with uterine fibroid tumors. You will reverse this somewhat when you are going through or have gone through menopause, a time when you are in need of estrogen. It's all about balance.

This means you must *read* labels, *even* the labels of your favorite *vitamins* to ensure the ingredients in them are not contributing to your challenge with uterine fibroid tumors and your cycle.

You must also *read* the *labels* and *inserts* on *prescription drugs* to ensure there are no possible adverse effects on your cycle. I read the insert of a prescription drug antihistamine that was given to me for an allergy, the insert said the drug could possibly cause "painful menstruation." WHO WANTS THAT? Of course, I said NO!

Microwaving, Aluminum and Plastics

(Other Things to Watch Out For)

- Go with a natural source for cooking your food, micro waving is out. Microwaving alters the molecules in food, especially water molecules, pulling the natural moisture out of food.

- Be careful when using aluminum— avoid direct and prolonged exposure of aluminum to food. It is being studied as a possible contributing factor to Alzheimer's disease. Aluminum can goods, cooking pots and pans and foil are some of the items falling into this category.

- Store (especially), drink and eat out of glass containers instead of plastic. Reason, estrogen-like substances are used in making some plastics.

Body Brushing

Body brushing helps remove impurities out of the body and is great for helping rid the body of *cellulite* (fatty, porous looking pockets on hips, thighs, arms and buttocks).

Purchase a body brush—a brush with a long handle and natural fibers on the end (some use a loofah). Before bathing brush all parts of your body in an upward motion towards your heart.

Herbal Bath

(Make Your Own)

Taking a natural herbal bath also helps to pull impurities out of the body.

Fill a bathtub with hot (as warm as comfortable for you) tub of water.

> *Add 1/4 cup of sea salt (the larger the grains the better) &*
>
> *1/4 teaspoon of your favorite naturally scented fragrance oil*

Relax, light some candles and enjoy.

On Becoming a Vegetarian

I am not trying to make vegetarians out of everyone, that is not my mission nor the mission of this book, but I am trying to raise the awareness of the powerful affect that food can have on the body.

Whatever works for you, giving you the results (short and long-term) you are looking for, do it, however, if something is not working for you—is not giving you the results you want, and YOU KNOW IT, you have a choice to do something different. Right?

If the food you are eating is having an adverse effect on your body, then it is time to make a change. No ifs, ands, buts about it.

We must become more **conscious**, and **conscientious**, meaning we **know** and then we **do better** concerning what we are choosing to put in and on our body, and what we are choosing to do to the rest of the planet. For instance, chickens are feed "growth hormones" to make them grow faster so they can get to the market- place faster for somebody to make money, money, money. Estrogen is a "growth hormone." Consume more chicken, consume more estrogen than you need or your body can healthily handle.

When you eat meat, you are eating a lot more than what you are really seeing. Not to mention the inhu- mane ways cows are often slaughtered. Such cows go through a shock before being killed. When something goes through a shock, chemical defenses are set up. Can you imagine eating meat that has been shocked! And, hopefully you are not eating it (meat) fried when you do. If you are, you are eating a dose of artery clog- ging grease. Your heart and all organs of the body need your arteries to pump and receive blood/nutrients through. Even the U. S. Department of Agriculture promotes food guidelines that include more grains, fruits and vegetables and less meat, dairy, fats, oils and sweets. (Food Guide Pyramid)

If you must eat meat (go with baked, broiled or boiled and drain the fat), *fish* is better for you. In fact fish is a brain food, especially salmon, because it is high in omega 3 oil, one of the necessary nutrients to enhance memory. Vegetarians can get their omega oils from consuming *flaxseeds*. I have already discussed exten- sively in this chapter the importance (and the "how to") of adding flaxseeds to your diet.

I am a vegetarian--a vegan (a vegetarian that does not eat dairy or eggs), but I feel the thing that made one of the biggest difference in my diet concerning the elimination of uterine fibroid tumors, and the crazy periods that came along with them, was the addition of flax-seeds to my diet to help balance my hormonal level of excess, unopposed estrogen. I know a set of twins, one is a vegetarian and one is not, they both had uterine fibroid tumors in their thirties. I also have other friends who have various eating habits and have had uterine fibroid tumors, particularly in their thirties and early forties. I suggest to them all---add flaxseeds to your diet.

I enjoy being a vegetarian. I do not feel I am missing out on anything. In fact I feel I am gaining quite a bit—it works for me. Many times I am told I look much younger than the number of years of wisdom (I call it) I have. Of course, I don't believe in the number thing anyway. Age is a mind set. I am quite an energetic person, too, who loves dancing. Becoming a vegetarian was a gradual process for me, not a "must do." I have learned, and still learning, to eat the things I enjoy eating, but eat them in their most natural states.

The Indole-3-Carbinol in Bok Choy, Broccoli, Cauli-flower, Kale, Mustard Greens and Turnips...raw or steamed (may be lost in cooking water)...lessens the risks of...uterine tumors 50%.

Joseph B. Marion, *The Anti-Aging Manual, Revised Second Edition*

(some paraphrasing/summarizing)

On this I say, **eat more vegetables**!

Stay away from caffeine. Use natural herbal teas (non-caffeine...read labels, some herbal teas have caffeine). *Chamomile tea* is good and is relaxing.

Stay away from chocolate, it contains caffeine. Use *carob* as an alternative.

Stay away from white flour products (the body has challenges trying to get rid of white flour products, they are believed to contribute to uterine fibroid tumors). Again, eat whole grain products instead.

Stay away from white rice, it is stripped of nutrients. Go with **brown rice** instead.

Herbal Seasonings
Good For You

Rosemary—B1, B3, calcium, manganese, C, potassium, *iron*, zinc, phosphorus, magnesium. Greenish/yellowish/grayish, bitter/minty.

Turmeric—B1, B2, B3, manganese, C, iron, potassium, calcium, phosphorus, zinc. Golden yellowish/orange, spicy.

Thyme—iron, B1, B2, B3, manganese, C, phosphorus, zinc, potassium, magnesium, amino acids, calcium, selenium and essential fatty acids. Light-medium green/strong husky, somewhat minty taste.

Cayenne Pepper—phosphorus, zinc, iron, C, E, amino acids, B1, B2, B3, B5, B6, folic acid, calcium, potassium and essential fatty acids. Deep reddish/orange, hot.

Garlic (powder or granulates)— selenium, calcium, potassium, magnesium, B1, B2, B3, phosphorus, manganese, iron, C and folic acid. Light yellowish/beige, aromatic.

Herbal seasonings can be purchased in bulk (less expensive & greater quantity) at health food stores and fresh fruit & vegetable markets, like *Farmers'* Markets. Purchase *organic* seasonings, no pesticides, artificial colorings or additives.

Don't use rosemary if you are pregnant.

Some Helpful Tips

- *Don't try to make all changes at once.* Slowly, but steadily make changes.

- *Keep a log* (length of your period, what worked, what did not work, etc.) of your cycles each month. If you have good results keep doing what you are doing, if not, make appropriate adjustments. For example, if you find that after eating fried food quite a bit over the last month brought on the results of a heavier period, cut back or stop eating fried food.

- *Be patient*, especially when first starting out on making positive changes. Most changes will take between three (3) and six (6) months to see. It takes about that long for a woman's hormonal make-up to change. Even if it takes you longer to see results, *be consistent.*

- Buy fruits and vegetables that are on sale. That is a good indication of what is in season (in abundance), saves you money and gives you variety.

- When exploring and learning on your own about the content and affects of food, supplements and the like, read from several different sources. Although this approach may be confusing at times, you will find that there is no one external source that has all the answers. Reference and cross reference the data. When you see something quite often, there you find a common ground. Hence, a possible answer.

Sample Menses Log

Date On	Days between last cycle	# of days on
May 16, year	27	5

Type of cycle:
2nd day medium/heavy, period gone by day 6

Comments:
-taking flaxseeds, one tablespoon twice a day
-pretty good eating habits this last month

June 9, year	25	7 plus light spotting 1 day after cycle

Type of cycle:
2nd day medium/heavy, lasted longer & one day spotting

Comments:
-ate a lot of fried food this last month
-constipated
-taking flaxseeds, some, but not daily
                                                    etc...

Illustration in sample is based on a person's results that has been consistent with a good basic natural diet, including flaxseeds, and little-to-no fried foods for quite some time (years). Each person's results are based upon that person's chemical makeup, diet and lifestyle.

When counting days between your cycle (actual flow), start counting as day one the first day of the actual flow of your cycle until the next day one of your actual flow. A typical cycle is around every 27-28 days, lasting seven days. Learn what is the healthy norm for you and monitor your norm. And, trust your intuitiveness in knowing when something is in or out of order concerning you.

> THE BEST WAY TO LEARN ANYTHING IS
> BY
> DOING/EXPERIENCING IT, THEN YOU
> KNOW FOR YOURSELF WHAT WORKS
> FOR YOU.

When I set out on this journey, I stop eating and putting anything on my body that I read increased the circulation of estrogen. And, I later started adding those items I read decreased the amount of circulating estrogen in the body. [I had read many times that it is believed uterine fibroid tumors are related to estrogen, considering that fibroids usually disappear after a woman goes through menopause.] Plus, during the period of time the tumors were releasing themselves from my body I had stopped taking vitamin supplements, I started to eat my vegetables (my vitamins). I also stopped taking soy protein supplements which I had been taking for a while (couple of years). On this note, now there is a lot of emphasis placed on adding soy to the diet. I am not so sure this is necessarily a good thing for women experiencing uterine fibroid tumors. Based upon my experience, I would say yes, soy (tofu, soy milk, primarily) is a good thing in moderation for women still in their menstruating years, and definitely as an alternative to meat. Nevertheless, soy has properties similar to estrogen, and is, therefore, perhaps more advantageous for women going through menopause to include in their diets more frequently (daily, etc.).

Summary

In this chapter dietary changes were addressed. The next chapter focuses on lifestyle changes.

By learning to contact, listen to, and act on our intuition, we can directly connect to the higher power of the universe and allow it to become our guiding force.

—Shakti Gawain—

5

LIFESTYLE CHANGES

Prayer
Meditation
Thoughts
Beliefs
Words—What are we telling ourselves?
Exercise, Walking
Joyous, Stress-Free living

Things that go on with us happen as a part of a total package—**mind, body and soul**. So, we must look at all of ourselves when addressing any aspect of our being.

Prayer

Prayer is when we connect with our Higher Source. It is a spiritual connection. It is when we purposefully turn toward The Divine—the all-knowing, all powerful Essence of Creation—for guidance.

Prayer is when we speak to God; remember the things to be grateful for; make our requests known; and go in peace knowing that all is well.

Meditation

Meditation is when we *listen to God.* It is the voice (some call it *intuition, wisdom...*) within that leads and guides us.

Meditation can be done while sitting quietly, taking deep breaths in and out; taking a walk...

watching a *sunset*

sitting before a *fireplace*

listening to *autumn leaves crunch*

lighting a *candle*

Or, just by simply *turning off* the *radio* in the *car.*

Thoughts, Beliefs and Words

Thoughts, beliefs and words help create our reality.

What are you telling yourself? Sitting around waiting to have fibroids and a hysterectomy because your mother and your grandmother had them is self-sabotage. If you think constantly that you will have to have an operation and speak the words, you probably will have to have an operation. Some believe in hereditary factors, but *some believe that what we think/believe about ourselves many times becomes our reality because we can't see anything else.*

Yes, heredity may play a part...the whole family make-up must be looked at. Sometimes it is just simply time to break the cycle of some things that have been passed along, maybe it is just time to stop the cycle (now that we know) of putting things in our food that may not be the best for us, like too much and the wrong kind of fat/oil. *Our ancestors did the best they could and knew at the time.* Now is the time for us to do the best that we can and know at this time.

If you are having a challenge with uterine fibroid tumors, along with dietary changes you must also examine your thoughts, belief systems and words surrounding the experience.

It is acknowledged here that for many reasons, sometimes medical, personal preference, etc. a hysterectomy or some other form of surgery may be the *solution* for someone. Work with your doctor.

Use **wisdom** in all your decisions.

Sometimes we have to give up old belief systems that are no longer serving us, replacing/affirming such belief systems with something better.

Affirm that you are healthy, whole and complete, even when you don't see the evidence yet that your body is healing. The mind is a very powerful tool. What the mind thinks, the body will follow. Therefore, make sure your mind is guided by a higher level of consciousness that knows the truth of your being—YOU ARE HEALTHY AND WHOLE.

Affirm

To *affirm* means to

> *approve*
>
> *claim*
>
> *assert*
>
> *state*
>
> *declare*

Go ahead approve, claim, assert, state, declare your healing. Believe it is possible for you to be well/healed.

Affirmation

(repeat three times with enthusiasm)

My Body is Whole and Healthy!

My Body is Whole and Healthy!

My Body is Whole and Healthy!

THINK healthy, BELIEVE it and SPEAK it, along with ACTIONS (good dietary and lifestyle choices/habits)

Faith and Actions

(as guided by the Holy Bible: James 2:14-18 & 24, the New Oxford Annotated Bible, with The Apocrypha, New Revised Standard Version)

Exercise

Exercise is a necessity. Try walking five (5) times a week, 20-30 minutes a day.

Don't exercise immediately after eating. Your body needs the energy to digest food. Wait at least two (2) hours before exercising after you have eaten a full course meal.

Joyous/Stress-Free Living

Practice joyous/stress-free living.

1. The first thing on the list in this category is to ensure you are in the correct job/profession— on the *correct career path*. Take some time to do some soul searching. The way you make a liv- ing—*your job/profession—should be in harmony* with *your desires* and *natural talents*.

   > [Suggested further reading, *Spirituality in the Workplace* and *How to Get Your Boss to Work for You*, by Faye Hardaway. Ordering informa- tion provided at end of this book.]

Any disharmony (dis-ease) in any aspect of your life, especially your job, the place where you spend a significant amount of your life, may contribute to disharmony/dis-ease in your body.

Correct your job/career choice to ensure balance in your life with the things most important to you, like family.

2. Do things that bring you inner joy, like listening to soft, comforting music; going to a spiritual service; sitting in the park; reading inspirational books, etc.

3. Join a yoga or some other class focusing on deep breathing and relaxation.

4. Take a relaxing herbal bath (ingredients given in the previous chapter on how to make your own herbal bath solution). Light some candles, *burn some incense* (*lavender* is good for helping emotions, *frankincense* and *patchouli* are also good) and relax.

5. Turn the telephone ringer off and *SLEEP*. There is no substitute—no vitamin, no medical pill that can take the place of a **good night's sleep**.

I was in a health food store one day when a lady in her mid thirties rushed into the store after work, talking particularly fast about how very *busy and tired* she was. She was looking for something to give her energy. I simply looked at her calmly and said, "sleep!" I proceeded to share with her that she already had the answer—she had stated she was "overworked." The lady smiled and said, "Thank you" and walked out the store. She wrote me later a much happier person. A simple answer for a seemingly big challenge. Life is just that simple. It is the simple things that make us happy, and they don't cost a penny. Keep it simple, listen to your own body and words. You have more answers than perhaps you think you do.

6. *Examine relationships, especially intimate relationships,* around you. (I have already spoken of relationships concerning your job/career, boss, co-workers, etc.) Those that are closest to you— a husband or a boyfriend—must be a positive addition to your life and not an extra burden, adding more stress. Stress equals dis-ease emotionally and physically.

Intimate relationship challenges—troublesome relationships, the wrong mate, being "unequally yoked" (having different interests, desires and aspirations and in some cases, differences in religions—approaches to life) and/or worrying about the lack of a husband or boyfriend to make one feel complete are probably some of the most common contributing factors to stress problems (imbalances) regarding uterine fibroid tumors. Examine your relationships!

Check out areas in your life where you might be emotionally holding on to an old hurt, or hurts, and LET GO.

Clean house in your relationships. This is not to point the finger externally. You must clean house internally, too. This is a very important part of overcoming uterine fibroid tumors. **Take some personal growth classes, read self-improvement books, join a good support**

group or see a counselor, if necessary. *Work daily on being the "best you" you can be.*

> *Acknowledge and address your emotions, they play a part in how your body responds.*

One of the books I find to be most instrumental in overcoming relationship challenges, whether it be husband, wife, boyfriend, girlfriend, mother, father, sister, brother, friend (or so called friend), etc. is *What You Think of Me is None of My Business* by Terry Cole-Whittaker.

> *Look for ways to express our creativity—a natural gift from God.*

7. Plan and prioritize the things you would like to accomplish. *You do not have to accept every requests* from others to help them with their top priority item. Learn to say, "No" sometimes, and stick with it. Women by nature are caregivers, sometimes forgetting to take care of themselves. You cannot help someone else most effectively when you are drained yourself. Take care of yourself and you will be better able to take care of others, i. e. share with others.

> Practice the art of just being *quiet* and *calm*.

Summary

Lifestyle changes are an integral part of your healing, they help tie the whole person together.

The next chapter is a sharing of my experiences as I went from doctor (medical and holistic) to doctor trying to find an answer to uterine fibroid tumors.

In prayer one must hold fast and never let go, because the one who gives up loses all. If it seems that no one is listening to you, then cry out even louder. If you are driven out of one door, go back in by the other.

—Jane Frances De Chantal—

6

My Story Continued

"If at first you don't succeed,
try, try again."

*Thomas H. Plamer, Teacher's
Manual [1840]*

te•na•cious

Holding or tending to hold
firmly; persistent;
holding fast

*The American Heritage Diction-
ary* s.v. "tenacious"

It had been a few months now. I was not satisfied with what the first doctor had told me ["We all have them...and will eventually have to have a hysterectomy...let's wait and see," she said].

My periods were not getting better or at least I was not comfortable with having the knowledge that something was wrong with my body. As they say, "What you focus on expands and grows."

I told a friend of mine about my experience at the first doctor's office. She told me about her doctor who she said was a specialist and was well thought of. She had gone to him for a pre-cancerous condition of the cervix that he had performed laser surgery on. She was pleased with him.

The second doctor's office had dark colors and the patients looked sad, unlike the first doctor's office which was decorated in bright, feminine colors and the atmosphere was upbeat. I found out the second doctor was an oncologist (specializing in the treatment of cancer).

As I was signing in the second doctor's office, another lady working at the same company as I (what a coincident, twice now) approached me and asked was this my first visit and which doctor I was there to see. When I told her which doctor, she almost jumped with joy. She told me that the doctor my friend sent me to see was also her doctor and that he (the doctor) was great. She went on to tell me that she had had the same pre-cancerous condition that my friend had had and that this particular doctor was doing her follow ups (she had to have pap smears every six months just like my friend). She said she was doing fine and her pap smears have been normal every since the surgery years ago.

This was all comforting, knowing that others felt highly of the new doctor I was about to see.

An assisting doctor was the person who actually examined me in this office and told me that I had fibroids. After the examination, he said get dress and the doctor you came to see will see you.

The second doctor was an older gentleman. When I told him of my frightening experience at the first doctor's office (the immediate idea of a hysterectomy being presented to me), he just laughed, shook his head as he called the first doctor's name that I had visited with amazement. Although he seemed to have thought highly of her, he thought she had "jumped the gun" too soon.

The older gentleman doctor said that I should have an exploratory, hysteroscopic procedure in which he would insert an instrument with a light through my vagina, take a closer look to see what the situation was and would remove any fibroids he saw...via scrapping my uterus. He also referred to a portion of the procedure as a D & C which people used to commonly get when my mother was experiencing challenges with her periods. This would have to be a surgery, but I would not have to be cut on the outside of my body and it would require that I check into the hospital for one day. It was an outpatient procedure.

Well, the procedure the second doctor performed did not work. He said that the fibroid tumor was not on the inside of my uterus so he could not shave it off. He went on to very tiredly tell me that he would have to give me Lupron to shrink the tumor, and then later do surgery— a myomectomy (abdominal) to remove the tumor. He said it would take 6 to 8 weeks to recover. I was now working in New York on a new, one year career advancement job assignment. I had just flown into Atlanta for my doctor's appointment. I told the doctor that I could not careerwise (in hindsight, what a reason—part of the problem...being overworked/stressed out) take 6 to 8 weeks off at this time.

I asked the second doctor what other options did I have and he gave me a pack of birth control pills and told me that some women find relief from their periods by taking birth control pills. I rushed back to Atlanta's Hartsfield International Airport to meet my boss and fly to Washington, D. C. for another business meeting the same day. I mentioned to my boss on the plane that the doctor said I might have to have surgery and it would take 6 to 8 weeks for recovery. He (*my boss*, a top executive) looked at me with a disappointing, wry smile and said, *"Women just have things that go on and get in the way,"* making reference to the *"unnecessary"* time to be spent *away from work*. WOW!

As I sat shocked and sad on the plane, I opened the inside reading material of the birth control pills the doctor had given to me and began to read.

I read *birth control pills could cause...*

blood clots

weight gain

liver tumors

increase the tendency to develop strokes

(the "stoppage or rupture of blood vessels in the brain")

death or serious disabilities

cancer of the reproductive organs

gall bladder disease

sharp chest pains

loss of vision

breast lumps

difficulty sleeping

jaundice or yellowing of the skin or eyeballs

severe headaches

vomiting

dizziness

fainting

heart attacks

fatigue

mood swings

irregular vaginal bleeding

melasma (dark patchy spots, especially on the face)

severe depression

To this I said, "NO."

So there I was in New York for a year working diligently (overworked) in my career, and hanging on as my bleeding got increasingly worse. During this time I became closer to becoming a vegetarian. However, I still was eating "junk food" to some extent, specifically potato chips cooked in the wrong type of oil. I now know better!

In hindsight some of the things I was advised to do, and did, in search for an answer/solution to uterine fibroid tumors were funny, downright ridiculous, but were all a part of a journey that led to a healing.

I went to over seventeen (17) doctors (including naturopaths), read countless books and articles, went to seminars, joined a support group, ate seaweed, had colonics, talked to many women, asked my mom and grandmother, sister, aunt, friends...God all to find an answer.

My upbringing is of the Christian Faith (Methodist). The Bible, our Holy book says,

"..Seek, and Ye Shall Find"

Matthew 7:7

> *"...For every one that asketh receiveth; and that seeketh findeth; and that knocketh it shall be opened."*
>
> *Matthew 7:8*

The *third doctor* was very mild mannered. At least, he took the time to explain to me the make up of uterine fibroid tumors—"(Noncancerous) S*mooth muscle* and *fibrous* (stringy, ropy, gelatin like—sticky, gummy, gluey) *connective tissue* that *grow from the muscle wall of the uterus*," he said. He showed me glossy, medical brochure type pictures of uterine fibroid tumors—and various locations they can grow in and outside the uterus. And, he was *honest*—he told me that even when removed, "They (uterine fibroid tumors) *can grow back.*" He checked my iron level, told me it was a little low, recommended an iron pill, and told me watching one's iron level was really important when challenged with uterine fibroid tumors, especially if excessive bleeding is the problem. One other neat thing about the third doctor was instruments were warmed before examining, showing some thought and consideration to the comfort of the woman/patient.

The *fourth doctor* was a naturopath. He had me take special herbal capsules he made, and had me to insert exceptionally large, handmade tampon like, herbal packs into my vagina at night. The packs were messy. In hindsight, I should have checked out this doctor's credentials more. I lost faith in this doctor—the naturopath—when one day as I was leaving his office, another potential client had just walked in inquiring of an advertisement for a weight loss program, and the doctor told the person to look at me that I had been a client of his and had lost a lot of weight. This was blatantly not true (I was already small when I came to him), so I knew I could not come back to this doctor. This is not to say that all naturopath doctors are dishonest (I obviously believe in a natural approach as demonstrated by the writing of this book), this is just an experience that I cannot omit. Dishonesty/false claims do not fit in any profession and is a terrible trick to pull on people suffering and in need of help.

I joined a *support group*--a wonderful experience to meet other women of many nationalities, faiths and professions with similar and sometimes much different and difficult experiences. Although I came to the support group after reading an article on uterine fibroid tumors in a major magazine, there were women in the support group who did not have fibroids, including the facilitator. We all quickly learned that fibroids were not our problem...that we had other emotional issues/hurts (often, but not only, relationship related) that needed to be addressed. How true! So, we sat around in a circle each week and discussed what was on our hearts and minds. This was helpful emotionally.

I went on a *macrobiotic diet* (ate seaweed, etc.). Although there were natural components of this diet, like eating brown rice, this diet was very uncomfortable for me—we were not supposed to eat fruit that was grown beyond a 250 mile radius from where we lived, so in my case bananas were not on the list—I was living in Atlanta, GA. (USA) at the time and we do not grow bananas. I craved bananas while on this diet.

I purchased a $250 book, went to a seminar packed with other women in search for an answer, among other things we were told of a process/technique to insert a glasslike egg on a string into our vaginas and practice squeezing, supposedly to strengthen our female organs. I even called the doctor [*the fifth doctor*] (who had been trained via the conventional medical approach in America, later turned to natural healing) responsible for the program, for a $75, 15 minute telephone consultation. She seemed tired and told me that I (and all of the other women) must not have been following the program right. She suggested some specific additional herbs for the excessive bleeding. None of this worked for me.

Other Things I Tried

I tried *colonics*. A colonic *is* an in depth/extensive, *enema like procedure* to help clean out your colon done by a professional—a trained person in the wholistic field. Many people in the wholistic health field say that all diseases begin in your colon, therefore, old impact waste must be removed. A total of 5 gallons of water (not all at once) is commonly used for one colonic session. Several sessions are usually scheduled. This may vary according to the client's needs and desires, and the practices of the person doing the colonic(s). I went for a few sessions. You can watch (debris as it comes out through a clear tube during a colonic, if you like). My colon was so empty there was nothing really to come out. I met one colonic professional (with beautiful skin) who told me she once had a tiny fibroid and starved it. She told me, "You have to starve it."

So, I tried starving it (the fibroid away) by *fasting*. I went on a *vegetable and fruit juice fast* and almost made it for a full seven days. I stayed in the bed the full time due to a lack of energy. I felt like I was starving myself. Some people are better able to fast. This was *not for me*.

I went to another (the *sixth doctor*) naturopathic doctor (who was just getting into a natural approach....later I heard that *he was previously an emergency room doctor who started trying natural approaches* (like high dosages of vitamin C) to heal his patients. He put me on a *supplemental/herbal cleansing program* that had *dong quai* (an estrogen promoter) in it. It made me bleed (spot). I stopped taking it immediately and gave it to my sister (for colon cleansing purposes) who did not have any fibroids. The supplement, with dong quai, made my sister bleed/spot, too. She also stopped taking it.

The *seventh doctor* was a doctor from the California area, naturopathic. He practiced a *method with sound* (*two silver metal*, pencil length objects that he *clanged together*), and put me on a colon cleansing program. He had a challenged case of sinus and was sneezing a lot.

The *eight doctor* was a woman doctor from California, speaking at a seminar at a church in the Atlanta, Georgia area (USA). Her specialty was *a natural product for menopause,* which seemed to have been effective for that purpose. She (the doctor) indicated that she was using the product herself with good results after trying and not desiring to be on synthetic hormone replacement therapy. After the seminar, I approached the doctor and personally talked with her about my challenge with uterine fibroid tumors. I asked her if the ingredients in the product would help with fibroids. She did not tell me that she did not know. She paused a moment and said, "I don't see why not." I later found out (through reading/further research on my own of each ingredient listed on the bottle) that the ingredients in the product were estrogen promoters, i.e. the product would give me more estrogen—the very thing I did not need more of. Besides, the product had valerian (a nervine, calmative type herb/tonic) in it and made me very sleepy. I could not take the fully prescribed amount and had to take it approximately 15 minutes before I wanted to go to sleep. The good thing about the product was that it was very relaxing. Relaxation is something highly stressed professional working (or homemakers) women going through menopause or challenged with uterine fibroid tumors can use. The product changed my hormonal level and gave me pimples, it was like I was a teenager again who had eaten chocolate (chocolate is something my dermatologist once told me I should stay away from to help avoid pimples when growing up). Nevertheless, I stopped taking the product because of its increasing estrogenic properties.

I also went to a *Chinese* doctor (the *ninth doctor*), briefly, who told me he did not have anything to treat uterine fibroid tumors.

The *tenth doctor* was a *chiropractor*. I could not adjust to the concept of that—the bending and pushing of the bones (the spine) into adjustment. I tried. There was only one adjustment that the chiropractor could give me (that I could allow/accept comfortably). It was an adjustment around the neck area, and I must say afterwards I felt exceptionally well relaxed (although my challenges with my cycles continued). As a child I recall my grandfather and grandmother going to a chiropractor and having good results. My grandmother is of 90 years of wisdom at the time of this writing. After giving me a urine test and finding blood (I was still spotting most of the time from the fibroid tumor), the chiropractor told me I had to get clearance from another medical doctor (in a different field) in order to continue with him (the chiropractor), which I did. I finally gave this up, too.

My bleeding was still heavy, so I conceded to going to the eleventh doctor.

The *eleventh doctor* said, "You must have a *myomectomy*"—fibroid to be removed (bikini line incision), uterus left intact, future conception of a child (or children) still possible, but may require C-section for delivery. I finally went along with this. I had a myomectomy. It did not work for me. I knew this immediately following the surgery. My next cycle was not only heavy, but now painful. I had to call the doctor on call within the first two weeks of the surgery—this doctor prescribed an anti-inflammatory medication (like, ibuprofen) to help curb the excessive bleeding. This did not work for me, either.

After going back to the doctor who performed my myomectomy for the six week check-up following the surgery, and telling her there was no change in my cycle, i.e. the bleeding was still very heavy, the doctor offered no explanation and I could not get back in to see her—she was "extremely busy" the nurse told me. So, I was left hanging. By the way, this doctor was related to a very large, ...reputable research hospital. I had excellent insurance and wanted the best, especially if I had to be cut on. Still I was left hanging, and to add to the frustration I was sent a $370 bill *three years later* and harassed by the billing department for an over $10,000 surgery that did not work which had already been paid for by my insurance company and I.

I told this to the administrative manager of the hospital and told her that if the doctor doing the surgery was too busy to see patients after their surgery, especially if there were problems, that she (the doctor) should consider not taking anymore patients until she has satisfactorily addressed/helped those who were already her patients.

I continued to bleed excessively for months after the myomectomy. It now took three months to get in to see the doctor following each visit or call. The doctor finally gave me some birth control pills which she said, "To control the bleeding." I gave in and took the birth control pills—my periods were now consuming too much of my life. I went from weighing 123 lbs. to 150 lbs. in seven months while taking the birth control pills and spotted (break through bleeding) the whole time. I was on my period for three weeks now and off for only one week versus the other way (normal) around.

My periods were now consuming too much of my life. I could feel blood gushing out, along with large clots dropping, especially when standing or sitting.

On airplane trips I was afraid I would mess up the seat on even an hour and a half flight to New York. I frequently went to the ladies room to check myself and to change my already "overnight" size pad. This was also true at work (in meetings) or church (one church I attended had white seats) or the movie theater, the park, during concerts, shopping, while on vacation, etc.

When asked by a doctor how I knew my periods were a problem, I responded, every since my cycles started in my mid-teens I never gave them much thought...they (my periods) came on and they went off. With uterine fibroid tumors my cycles were now consuming too much of my time.

This was true for other women, too. I found out by talking with other women (my friends, etc.) that many of their problems with fibroids began in their early-to-mid thirties [some as early as their late twenties], a time when estrogen is considered to be "unopposed" by a decline in the progesterone level in a woman's hormonal cycle.

Some of my friends were told by their doctors that they were "perimenopausal" during this phase.

Perimenopause basically meaning the time preceding menopause.

Eldred B. Taylor, M.D., obstetrician/gynecologist, has spent considerable focus on understanding the various dynamics of fibroids, perimenopause and other common gynecological problems. I heard Dr. Taylor say in a seminar once he made the mistake of listening to a patient and that was one of the best mistakes he could have made. Out of that came a workable solution for the patient (combining efforts of the doctor and the patient) and led to education for other women on how their bodies function from a hormonal standpoint. *Dr. Taylor is an example of a medical doctor who is open enough to listen to his patients, go further than what has been traditionally known and, thereby, be of better service to his patients and beyond.*

Coincidentally (or maybe not, for those who believe there are no coincidences...only divine planning and timing), the woman being referenced was challenged with uterine fibroid tumors and was exploring/using a natural alternative (although different from the one described in this book). Dr. Taylor was not turned off by this, he listened.

Symptoms with fibroids can last until the mid-to-late forties, or until a woman goes through menopause.

Menopause means 12 consecutive months without a period, so it is the 1st year anniversary of your last period. I feel women should celebrate menopause with a party, especially when you consider how much we have complained of our periods. In fact, I feel each stage (the starting and stopping of menstruation) should be acknowledged, embraced [rites of passage] and celebrated.

The average age for menopause is 51 (for a woman in the United States) per most sources, like the FDA Consumer and Women's Health Weekly, but as with many things, things are changing—diets, lifestyles, etc. And, each woman is different. I know of one woman whose periods stopped naturally around 43 and another at 47, and yet, I know of a woman whose cycle was still on at 51 and an aunt who chuckled as she told me her cycle did not stop until she was 56, and another woman, of whom my mother told me about, who was in her sixties before her periods stopped. One internet source (Family Health Resources, ivillagehealth) reported a range of 48-55.

The menopausal cycle and associated symptoms (unpredictable periods coming on and off at various times of the month and sometimes not at all for several months, night sweats, hot flashes, etc.) experienced by some women vary. I know women who experienced no challenges at all with menopause. The same is true for uterine fibroid tumors.

As I mentioned previously, I was left on my own by the eleventh doctor, the one performing the myomectomy (to remove the fibroid)—the surgery that did not work for me. **I knew** something was still wrong and I kept inquiring of the doctor...I kept telling her something was still wrong..., and she just ignored me and said you need to go on birth control pills to control the bleeding...and said bye, basically released me.

The eleventh doctor had written on my chart "Very Knowledgeable." And I was. I had read many books and articles, anything I could get my hands on, about the so called dis-ease I (and thousands of other women) was challenged with called uterine fibroid tumors. So, when the morning nurse came in following my surgery (myomectomy) and asked how was I doing after a hysterectomy, I immediately responded, "That was not what I was supposed to have." So she went back out of the room, read my chart, came back in and said, "Oh yeah, you had a myomectomy."

Two students of the research hospital and school came into my room with amazement to talk to be about my being a vegetarian, particularly "vegan"—a vegetarian who does not consume dairy products or other animal by products, such as eggs. The students had found out I was vegan via my menu selection, of which was very limited in choices of quality food via the hospital's menu. The students asked me a lot of questions, went away... researched and came back to ask me more questions. For example, they wanted to know how I got vitamins B-12 and B-6—some things vegetarians are to ensure they get beyond animal sources. I told them how I got these two vitamins, basically through supplements at the time. They pleasantly smiled and went away.

> *I think the two medical students had a personal interest in becoming vegetarians. Surprisingly, I was later charged for "research on vegetarianism" by the hospital, of which I rightfully opposed since I was the one asked the questions. The charges came off my bill.*

> *It is interesting that the hospital, a place which should know better and is supposed to assist as patients get well, would serve "junk food" (food knowingly unhealthy for human consumption and create a lot of health challenges, many of which bring people to the hospital such as high blood pressure, heart diseases [clogged arteries....from eating too much fat—the wrong kind of oil in the diet, etc.]).*

At some point I had a *dream*. This goes back to women listening to their own intuition. In the dream, the dream very clearly said, "It's still in there." "It" being the uterine fibroid tumor. The dream was so profound it woke me up.

So, now back and forth to the doctor, whenever I could get in. Remember, I was now being told this doctor (the eleventh one, yes the one who performed the myomectomy on me that did not work) was so busy— "You are looking at three months before you can get in there," was the standard answer. I finally decided to see another covering doctor (the *twelfth doctor*). It was easier to get an appointment in this case. The covering doctor, the twelfth doctor, listened attentively and told me that *uterine fibroid tumors usually come in clusters, like grapes* and that the previous doctor probably did not get them all/particularly the one(s) causing the problem.

As a part of the routine office procedures, an attendant had me to weigh prior to seeing the doctor. I was alarmed. I weighed almost 30 pounds more than I had before the sixth doctor put me on birth control pills to "control the bleeding" 7-8 months ago. I told the attendant something must be wrong—I questioned whether or not the scale was right. The attendant did not take me seriously. She acted as though she thought I was being overly focused on my weight and told me, "Oh everybody says that about those scales."

Very concerned, I informed the twelfth doctor (the covering doctor) of the weight gain. I told her if it is not the scales then I believe the birth control pills have made me gain the weight. I checked myself on another scale independent of the doctor's office. It was not the scales, I had gained the weight while on birth control pills. I called the doctor's office and the doctor changed the pills to a smaller dosage—the mini pill—I believe. This still did not work for me—no relief—still long, heavy periods with spotting in between cycles. Three weeks on, one week off menses.

I had to ask for an ultrasound to see if a uterine fibroid tumor was still there. And when I took the ultra sound the ultra sound person was kind enough to tell me so because I had an "inquiring mind"...I looked on the monitor and she pointed them (two uterine fibroid tumors) out to me. Hence, I went back to the doctor (or at least via telephone via her nurse...this was still the eleventh doctor, the one leaving me hanging after the myomectomy). I started doing more and more reading. I asked the doctor to give me some *natural progesterone pills*, which she knew nothing about and finally reluctantly gave/prescribed them for me. She did not even know how to prescribe them. I found out the information and passed it on. And, I tried that—I took the natural progesterone pills. One learning experience about this was I had read the dosage must be monitored or you could have a headache. At one particular point in time I had the worst headache of my life, but it was also at a time after being told some very stressful news about a classmate whose brother had murdered him. Nevertheless, at any rate, this is just another reminder for women to listen to your own intuition and "Seek, and Ye Shall find" (Holy Bible, Matthew 7:7).

During recovery after I had the myomectomy, I could hear and see a nurse in my room on the telephone telling someone that I was "orange". It is amazing how the mind works even when you are going through recovery after undergoing anesthesia. I knew that I had been drinking carrot juice and that carrot juice over a period of time could give you somewhat of an orangish looking tint. So, still heavily sedated, I sleepily told the nurse, "It's carrot juice."

I had been so strong, for so many months and years with the challenge of uterine fibroid tumors, however, in the prep room of the operating area in which I had my myomectomy I broke down and cried. The last thing I wanted was to be cut on, and the attending nurse was having difficulty getting the IV tube in my arm. The anesthesiologist came in and very empathetically asked me what was wrong. I just cried and he looked so sadden by my tears. He went ahead and gave me something to calm me down (and it did...it put me to sleep) before having the nurse to continue.

On the drive home after a five day stay in the hospital for the myomectomy, I was happy (optimistic that this would work....would solve all my problems, I hoped). Approximately a mile away from the hospital my mother had to stop the car. I felt like something had been taken out of my stomach area, leaving an empty space. I was nauseated by the car ride and the least bump in the road felt like my organs in the lower part of my stomach were bouncing around. So, more tears. Some expressing a feeling of relief (I had been through so much) and some expressing a feeling of discomfort from the ride. My grandmother was riding in the back seat, giving words of encouragement and my mom was doing the same in the front seat as she drove me home. Thanks God for mothers and grandmothers, and all the women who have gone before us with this challenge.

The incision for the myomectomy was straight across my belly about 6 inches long. I was Bent over for several weeks after the surgery. I wondered if I would ever stand up straight again. I did! That's another blessing. The recovery time was six-to-eight weeks. My mom stayed with me during this time. I had a few stairs in my home I had to be concerned with.

Even though I was very careful, somehow I pulled a stitch a loose, and some bleeding started from the incision. Of course I felt a little discouraged that day, but I called the doctor and was told this was nothing to worry about...I was instructed to clean the incision and to put some bandage strips across the area. This worked fine.

I had to buy new underwear because that "bikini line" cut the doctor said she would give me was exactly on the panty line of my current undergarments and was quite irritating.

To top it off, I was constipated, before and after the surgery. Constipation is something common with some women experiencing uterine fibroid tumors. This added to my concern for not wanting to disturb the stitches from straining.

I was getting nowhere with the current doctor, so it was time to move on. I took myself off the birth control pills and did just that—moved on.

Each woman's experiences are different—uniquely her own. Some women have had myomectomies with good results.

I have a girlfriend who had a myomectomy, re-started with a different brand of birth control pills afterwards and has had no additional problems with her periods or reoccurring fibroids. She is 47 now.

This same friend (let's call her Alice) had an experience in which a doctor told her he did not believe in myomectomies, that she (the patient) could either have a hysterectomy or nothing at all. Alice says she found out that sometimes those who have not experienced the problem (and I add here, male or female) can be insensitive. She laughed as she told me she had 5 second opinions before finally deciding on a doctor.

Alice was only bent over for a couple of days following her mymomectomy versus my few weeks, however, her full recovery period was still six-to-eight weeks before she was able to go back to work.

I met a lady in the hospital who after five years of no problems was having her second myomectomy (the fibroids grew back). She was 45, and newly married, at the time of her second surgery. Her brother (a medical doctor) told her, "Whatever you do, don't let them give you a hysterectomy...there are just too many complications afterwards and there are other alternatives."

The *thirteenth doctor* I visited was kind, listened to my whole history with uterine fibroid tumors, and was careful not to suggest a hysterectomy. Only one problem, he kept giving me pap smears (which came back slightly abnormal) when I had clearly told him I was still spotting from my cycles. This created extra worry and resulted in my having to go and have a small in diameter chunk of my uterus removed for testing. This was painful, but I am grateful the test was done. It is best to check many avenues. All was well. My challenge was still a uterine fibroid tumor.

I found out a girlfriend's doctor gave her Provera (medroxyprogesterone acetate, a progestin [synthetic progesterone]) to cut her periods off each month at the end of her cycles because she was on a blood thinner and her blood would not clot/stop in this case. So, I thought maybe this could help me with the excessive bleeding related to uterine fibroid tumors. I asked my doctor if I could try this medication. He said o.k., but told me, "It is not going to work." I tried it, I even had the doctor to increase the dosage to the same level my friend was receiving. No luck. It did not work for me.

The doctor suggested "we" (I like that—a patient/doctor team approach) try something like Depo-Provera (another type progestin, i. e. synthetic progesterone) which would be given in shot form once a month. He said some people use this method for birth control purposes and it might cause the period to go away, which could be helpful to someone experiencing excessive bleeding during cycles (as in the case with uterine fibroid tumors). When I asked of the side effects of this approach, the doctor said, "1% of the people complain of thinning hair." Although a small percentage...well, who wants that challenge? I said, "No" to this approach.

My *thirteenth doctor* took a *leave of absence*. I had to go to another doctor during this period of time for my routine pap smear.

When telling her, the *fourteenth doctor*, of my challenges (still on-going) with uterine fibroid tumors, she very sternly said, "**You have to have a hysterectomy**."

I had a list of questions already made out in an effort to not take up too much of the doctor's time. I asked about a procedure called endometrial ablation—a procedure in which the lining (the part that bleeds/sheds each month) of the uterus would be cauterized (burned away with a hot balloon/rollerball). She told me that she did not know how to do this procedure, but knew someone who did, and I would have to take something like Lupron (a GnRH agonist) or DepoProvera (a progestin) prior to the procedure/surgery in order for the procedure to be more effective. I have already discussed GnRH agonists and progestins. The reason for taking such medication first (prior to the endometrial ablation procedure) is to decrease the build up in the endometrial— lining of the uterus.

The Hysterectomy Educational Resources and Services (HERS) Foundation, an organization dedicated to sharing information about the consequences of hysterectomy and alternatives, was helpful in sending me more information on the procedure.

And, I called and asked another doctor willing to provide information over the telephone. He told me that with a _endometrial re-section_ or _ablation_ there was:

-zero chance of having children

(although you keep your uterus)

-60% reported no bleeding

(no actual flow of menstruation)

-20%-35% reported periods/menstrual

bleeding not as bad

-5% failure rate (did not help)

I also spoke with a woman (a friend of mine) who had had the surgery/procedure—endometrial ablation. She was about 10 years older than I. She said she had not had any problems/complaints after the procedure. She said her periods had completely gone away after the surgery. She was now experiencing a strong case of menopause challenges (frequent hot flashes which kept her fanning most of the time and her face wet with moisture), she does not contribute this to the endometrial ablation procedure, just mother nature.

Complaints I had Heard and/or Read
about Hysterectomy

loss of energy

vaginal dryness

bladder challenges

depression

weight gain

loss of feeling of sensuality, and others

One girlfriend of mine told me that her doctor (a male doctor of whom she trusted) told her, "If you have one—a hysterectomy you better not let your male friend know. Some men have hang-ups about this," he said. Although interestingly, he told her that his wife had had a hysterectomy. We (women and men) have a lot to learn and release about this.

I must say here that I have **also known women who say they have had absolutely no problems after a hysterectomy**. Some have felt relieved from the heavy cycles that were created previously by the presence of uterine fibroid tumors. And, I have known of women who have asked for a hysterectomy even before one was suggested/recommended by their doctor. I know of a woman who asked her GYN for a hysterectomy after having her last child (the doctor refused the request because there was nothing wrong with her uterus— she did not have fibroids at the time). However, this same lady said the first time her doctor detected the presence of a fibroid, she (the patient) asked for a hysterectomy.

As I have said previously each woman's experiences and desires are different. We as women must *honor our wisdom within* for what is best for us individually. The best that we can do for each other is provide loving SUPPORT.

111

When telling her, the fourteenth doctor, of my *concerns* and *fears* relating to not wanting to have a hysterectomy (not wanting to lose my capacity to have children—I had never been married or had children yet, and had read horrible things about the after effects some women experience after a hysterectomy, such as loss of sex drive, etc.), she said, "**YOU NEED TO GROW UP**!" "I need to have one too. Now let's schedule it (yours)." Wow!

Amazing Grace!

The *fourteenth doctor* **scheduled** a **hysterectomy** supposedly for me **October 26th**.

I knew a hysterectomy was not for me. I told everyone I talked with as a part of the surgery scheduling process, and the doctor, that this was just not for me—I was not a good candidate for this type of surgery—I had too many issues/concerns with it, primarily I did not want to lose a body part (my uterus) and lose my capacity to have children.

The doctor did not want to hear all of this.

*So, I went with the flow/the program externally and cried out in a different way. **I called upon my faith.***

Lying across my bed one day I just cried my heart out.

"...I cried upon the Lord and He heard me."
Psalm 120:1

I knew within my heart and soul that there had to be a better way—that women should not have to endure such. I followed my intuition—the wisdom within.

On **Oct. 5th** of that same year, **I called the doctor's office** and **asked for the surgery** (the scheduled hysterectomy) **to be cancelled** and moved/**rescheduled one month later**. The surgery was rescheduled for Dec. 6th, pre-op with the doctor was to take place Nov. 30th.

On Oct. 13, nine days after I had cancelled the first scheduled surgery, the uterine **fibroid tumors** were **releasing themselves** naturally from my body. NO NEED FOR A HYSTERECTOMY!

Hallelujah, the power of prayer—thought—faith.

This cannot be ignored by the medical profession and should not be ignored by you, either, as you consider your desires for a happy and healthy life, as reflected earlier in the chapter of this book on lifestyle changes and the *power of your thoughts, words and belief system.*

I did my part, too. I educated myself on what was going on with me and what I could do to help myself. I read, read, read. Then I went into action. I changed my diet to take out those things (given to you in this book previously) that would bring me discomfort/disease...uterine fibroid tumors and I added those things which would make things better for me.

Just as you can't desire apples and plant oranges, you can't put the wrong things in your body and expect good menses. Your monthly menstruation is another way the body releases itself.

It is amazing (amazing grace) what faith and a small seed (in this case, a flaxseed), can do. Nature has all we need. If we will just take heed and stop accepting—buying into the idea that money, money, money is the most important thing at any cost (packing foods with harmful growth hormones, pesticides, etc.), even at the expense of human health.

Faith and Actions

It was not always easy for me to give up things that I had grown to like, like potato chips (cooked in the wrong oil—hydrogenated—or high in saturated fat content). It was about knowing better, then doing better. I gradually changed. Much of eating is out of habit. Habits can be changed. I gave up one version of food for another version. For example, if I want a healthy sweet snack, I now know if I choose to, I can have raisins and raw almonds and be satisfied versus a sugary candy bar that has a lot of things in it that will not get me the results I want. Or, I can choose corn chips cooked in cold pressed canola oil, etc. There are unlimited food choices that one can make and be satisfied and healthy.

The thirteenth doctor returned. I went to him for a routine pap smear—his office was closer.

When being checked, the doctor yelled, "I see what your problem is...THERE IS A UTERINE FIBROID TUMOR TRYING TO DELIVER ITSELF!"

> *I responded, "So, what do we do now?" The doctor said, "I don't know.............let's wait and see what happens."*

THIS WAS A BIG BREAKING/DISCOVERY POINT

When my cycle came on the next time, a couple of weeks later, it was flowing heavy as usual with the fibroids. Only this time when I sat on the toilet, as large clots and a stream of blood was gushing out (again, an experience I was used to with uterine fibroid tumors), I felt an urge to push. I could feel something lodged in my vagina area. I examined myself and could feel *something solid, but soft.* I then grabbed a handheld mirror and looked. There I could see the *uterine fibroid tumor on its way out.* I had seen what one looked like via a picture a girlfriend of mine had of hers after a myomectomy. It *looked like a boiled egg* to me, but more round.

> *I CALLED THE THIRTEENTH DOCTOR, HE ASKED, "CAN IT WAIT?" I SAID, "NO!" HE CALLED THE OTHER DOCTOR (THE FOURTEENTH ONE) WHO IN TURNED CALLED ME AND SAID, "MEET ME AT THE EMERGENCY ROOM." THEY BOTH MET ME THERE IN AMAZEMENT.*

I was so excited and relieved all the way there. My mom, sister and grandmother took me to the hospital. No one at the hospital's emergency room believed what was happening—that the uterine fibroid tumor was releasing itself from my body.

The fourteenth doctor examined me, and said, "Yes a fibroid is trying to come out on its own." She looked at me with surprise and asked, making a statement at the same time, "You're not in any pain?" I replied, "No." The doctor said, "That's amazing. Usually when women are expelling fibroids in such a manner there is excruciating pain and they complain of a strange odor. You have none of that." She used the terminology "prolapsed cervical myoma" in explaining some of the dynamics of the occurrence. Myoma is another name for uterine fibroid. It was right at the opening of my vagina on its way out. To be on the safe side, the doctor said I would be taken to the operating room and she would snip it [the doctor said it turned out to be two, one smaller one attached to another one—like a "snowman"]. My mother told me it took approximately 15 minutes and I was out of the operating room, and my grandmother and aunt missed it because they had gone to get a quick bite to eat. The next time they saw me I was ready to be released. My mom said I asked the nurse could I get another little nap before I left the hospital and the nurse said, "Yes." I got my nap and we left the hospital the same day.

> *Now the same doctor who had told me (almost in-sisted) that I would have to have a hysterectomy almost a month ago was looking down at me in the emergency room and saying, "This could be it...this could solve your problem." And, it did. "There is no need for a hysterectomy," this same doctor said.*
>
> *I am grateful.*

The Natural Way

NO PAIN

NO INCISIONS

NO LONG RECOVERY PERIOD

  ONLY GRATITUDE!

All went well. I was happy. My periods were fine for a long time.

THE SECOND NATURAL RELEASING OF UTERINE FIBROID TUMORS

About two years later after my first experience with uterine fibroid tumors releasing themselves from my body, my monthly flow started being heavier (but no clots this time) for about six months.

I had started using a natural progesterone cream in an effort to possibly prevent uterine fibroid tumors from developing in the future. I had my *hormone levels checked* via a *saliva test* (proper name *Post-Menopausal Hormone, Short*)...I call it the "spit test" because you have to spit in a glass test tube type container. It was explained to me via a review of the results of the test that I now had too much progesterone in my system and that too much would give you the same effects as before...not having enough. So, the doctor instructed me to come off the progesterone cream for a while which I did. My flow was still messy/heavy, so **I started back on a regimen of what had worked for me before.**

[Note: One interesting thing I found out via the saliva test is that there are three types of estrogens in our hormonal makeup, estrone, estradiol and estriol. The doctor explained to me that estriol is the "good estrogen," therefore, it is o.k. for estriol to be on the high side. Of course they are all good when they are in the proper range for the individual's body.]

Each time I asked myself what was I doing differently when the fibroids were naturally releasing themselves (I had kept detailed records), the answer was I had incorporated *flaxseeds* (**two tablespoons a day**— one, twice a day) into my diet. This handled the excessive estrogen level side of the equation with uterine fibroid tumors. I was consistent...I did this—the total program—*physical* [example: adjusting my eating habits, exercising, etc.], *mental* and *spiritual*, over six-to-eight months and I still do it every day. It worked/and still works for me and I hope and pray it works for you, and all the other women experiencing the challenge of uterine fibroid tumors, too. I am free of this challenge and desire the same for others.

I found out I needed to balance the estrogen side. I read, read, read and I found that the properties of flaxseeds and a host of other things (shared with you in this book) could possibly do this. **On my own I had to learn how much to use, how often and how to process/prepare and consume flaxseeds to help my situation. This I shared with you in chapter 4.**

Part of the Journey

One beautiful hot, sunny Atlanta day while out riding I noticed a Mercedes Benz car dealership. I had been looking for a replacement car since I had lost mine back during the winter sliding on "black ice" (ice you don't know is there that is covering the black pavement) and crashing into, of all things, a tow truck.

On this particular sunny day I went onto the parking lot of the car dealership and picked out a beautiful silver toned light blue Mercedes with matching leather interior. I got in the car with the dealership's manager. He showed me the features of the car. We talked. I got out of the car, felt a little wet at the seat of my pants, looked down inside the car and noticed a big splash of blood from my cycle had spilled over on this silver <u>light blue</u> interior of the Mercedes. I was so embarrassed, but there was no time for that. I did the queenly thing. I told the gentlemen that I noticed I messed up his car seat, went on to tell him that I had some wipes in the car and I would take care of it. I cleaned up the mess and left the dealership. That was the last day I believe I looked at Mercedes. I bought an all purpose sports utility vehicle (SUV) instead.

I went straight to my mom's house to change clothes. I was just soaked with blood. The heavy flow of my cycle had gone through the heavy-duty/overnight size sanitary napkin I had on. I felt no pain, just shame. Yet, I know better than that. There was nothing to be ashamed of or embarrassed over, only a challenge to be released.

FIND A GOOD DOCTOR—one who will **listen** to you, **work with you**, and **along with your own intuition/wisdom**.

I was home again when the second natural releasing of uterine fibroid tumors was occurring. Again, I felt like something was lodged in my vagina area. I felt no pain, no discomfort, just a knowing that something was different. Again, as with the first releasing I examined myself (women know your body) and felt a similar solid, yet soft substance. Having gone through this before, I called the doctor—the one performing the previous clipping for safety reasons. I was told this doctor (the fourteenth one) was about to get off work and that I should go to the emergency room at the hospital and see the covering doctor.

When I got to the hospital, again my mom, sister and grandmother accompanied me, no one (the intake nurse, receptionist, on staff emergency room doctor nor the on call gynecologist) at the hospital believed what I was telling them—that a uterine fibroid tumor was releasing itself from my body. Even though I explained to them that this had happened before, and at the same hospital, still no one believed me.

The intake nurse said, "Oh, honey that never happens to anyone." I said, "Well, how about twice. Twice I have had uterine fibroid tumors to naturally start releasing themselves from my body." The intake nurse replied, "You must be pregnant." And she proceeded to type what she believed in the computer—that I must be pregnant.

The emergency room doctor (the fifteen doctor) was kind. She and I had a very good rapport. She was a middle aged lady and seemed to have been a seasoned doctor. She did not believe me either, even after an ultra sound that proved what I was saying—that a uterine fibroid tumor was trying to release itself from my body. Finally she told me, "Let me examine you and see for myself." She did—examined me—then looked at me with amazement, but conviction, and said, "You are right, a uterine fibroid tumor is trying to release itself." "I'm going to have your HMO's on-call gynecologist to come and look at you." [HMO is a type of health insurance and means Health Maintenance Organization. It functions as a large business corporation in the healthcare field.]

The on-call emergency room gynecologist (the sixteenth doctor) came in and said he was exhausted, he had just completed a surgery. He examined me, confirmed what I had been saying and what the ultra sound showed and told me that he was too exhausted to handle it this evening, I would be admitted into the hospital overnight and the on-call gynecologist (the seventeenth doctor) for the next morning would handle it—ensure that the fibroid is safely delivered. I know my boundaries. There are times when the skill/knowledge and wisdom of a doctor is needed (and greatly appreciated).

The on-call evening doctor (gynecologist) told me that I should be conducting seminars on the subject of uterine fibroid tumors and natural healing.

The emergency room doctor (general practitioner) said, "You really have the propensity to create these things (meaning fibroids)." I replied, "No I really have the propensity to get rid of them." This reminds me of the saying/question, "Is the glass half full or half empty?" I could only see the beauty of the releasing.

Nurses Inquiring of the Natural Approach

That night at the hospital from 10:00 p.m. until the wee hours of the morning two nurses stayed in my room inquiring of me of what I was doing differently resulting in uterine fibroid tumors releasing themselves naturally. I told them. They, too, were experiencing challenges with fibroids and said they had never seen anybody who was naturally releasing them. I said, "How about twice?" I encouraged them to keep the faith and watch their diets so they, too, could rid themselves of such a challenge. Another good thing about the whole process is that what I share in this book is not only good just for eliminating uterine fibroid tumors or just for women, but many components of it (a whole person approach), like eating healthy, good food and taking care of your emotions and spiritual side can be used by all people.

The next morning when it was time to go into the surgery room for the morning on-call gynecologist (the *seventeen doctor* I had seen throughout my experience with uterine fibroid tumors, and now the releasing) to assist with the uterine fibroid tumor naturally releasing itself, the morning on-call doctor walked into the room (she had never seen me before), looked at me (in the face...no examination) and sarcastically said, *"You need to go ahead and have a hysterectomy."* **I looked at her (the doctor) and looked around the room—my mother, grandmother, aunt and sister (three generations of women) were all sitting there. I then looked back at the doctor and firmly, but politely, said, "No." The uterine fibroid tumor was already releasing itself naturally. I went on to say, "Would you please just clip the fibroid that is coming out via my vagina, like the doctor did before, and let me go home." It was as though I was speaking for three generations of women, and all those before, two generations of which I know had lost their uteruses to hysterectomies because of uterine fibroid tumors. IT WAS TIME FOR THIS CYCLE OF HANDLING WOMEN IN THIS WAY TO STOP—NO MORE HYSTERECTOMIES for the cause of uterine fibroid tumors to be routinely handed out**. I was so happy my mother, grandmother, aunt and sister were sitting there. I gave them another look and said confidently to them, make sure under no circumstance she (the doctor) does a hysterectomy. My family looked back at me with confidence and assurance, no words were said or needed at this point. I knew they would look out for me and all the women of the world. *My aunt* said, "Let's pray." She *led the prayer*. The doctor was still there. *"God we know you will take care of _____. Thank you for letting this tumor naturally start releasing itself. Thank you for this doctor who has showed up this morning. Let this procedure be a success. We ask that you work through the doctor's hands. We know all is well. Thanks*

God. Amen" Then she said to the doctor, "Now you can take her...see you when you get back."

The seventeenth doctor was a Hispanic lady, suggesting a hysterectomy. I hope that no other culture of women, or women anywhere, of any race have to undergo such giving up of a body part (the seat of creativity in this case) that God made perfectly whole and healthy.

I don't know why this doctor was so quick to suggest a hysterectomy, when in this case it was clearly not needed. Maybe it was a money issue she thought for the insurance company/the HMO. Maybe that was her training. I don't know her reasoning, but what I can share is that from a cost standpoint to the insurance company both times the uterine fibroid tumors were releasing themselves naturally from my body, the cost for the overseeing and assistance from the doctors was cheaper for both times combined than for the myomectomy. It was a savings. And, besides I pay dearly monthly for the medical insurance coverage. In America such coverage is high. That is something that is being worked on in America to make better for people.

When I went back for the two week follow-up visit with the doctor, she walked in the room looked at me and said, "You are o.k....you can go."

The procedure the doctor did assisting with the delivery of the fibroid was a success and quick. I went home the same day with **no more challenges with uterine fibroid tumors**. THANKS GOD. I AM SO GRATEFUL.

Now, let me tell you about the greatest physician, the healer.

When at night you cannot sleep, talk to the Shepherd and stop counting sheep.

—Anon.—

7

THE RESULTS
"COMPLETION"

"Woman Your *Faith* Has Made You Whole"
Holy Bible, Luke 8:48

Natural cycle 7 days

The number 7 represents completion (healing)

There is a story in the Christian faith that deals with a woman with an *issue of blood* and *by her faith* she was made whole.

I feel as though I know this lady—I can certainly relate to her.

And there was a woman in the crowd who had an issue of blood for twelve years. She had spent all she had on physicians and could not be healed of any. She came behind Jesus (Yeshua, Jesus' Hebrew name) and touched the hem of his garment. Immediately the bleeding stopped.

"Who touched me?" Jesus asked.

Everyone denied it, and Peter (a disciple) said, "Master, this whole crowd is pressing up against you."

But Jesus told him, "No, someone deliberately touched me for I felt healing power go from me." When the woman realized that Jesus knew, she began to tremble and fell to her knees before him. She declared unto him before the whole crowd for what cause she had touched him, and how she was healed immediately.

And he said unto her, "Woman (Daughter most translations) your faith has made you whole; go in peace."

Luke 8:43-48
(paraphrasing)

Thanks God. And So It Is!

References & Other Information

References

Balch, Phyllis A., C.N.C. and Balch, James F., M.D., *Rx Prescription for Cooking & Dietary Wellness* (Revised), copyright 1992 by Phyllis Balch, C.N.C. and James Balch, Jr., M.C., F.A.C.S., PAB Books Publishing Co., Greenfield, Indiana.

Balch, Phyllis, A., CNC and Balch, James F., M.D., *Prescription for Nutritional Healing*, Third Edition, copyright 2000 by Phyllis A. Balch, published by Avery, A Member of Penguin Putnam Inc., New York, NY.

Baron-Faust, Rita, *Being Female*, What Every Woman Should Know About Gynecological Health, copyright 1998 by Rita Baron-Faust, William Morrow and Company, Inc., New York, N. Y.

Cole-Whittaker, Terry, *What You Think of Me is None of My Business*, copyright 1979 by Terry Cole-Whittaker, Jove edition, April 1988, Jove Books (published by The Berkley Publishing Group), New York, N. Y.

From preparation to recovery...understanding hysterectomy, An informative guide for women who have been advised to undergo hysterectomy or related surgery, 109-40621-A 2, copyright 1994 by Ciba-Geigy Corporation.

Marion, Joseph B., *The Anti-Aging Manual*, The Encyclopedia of Natural Health, Revised Second Edition, copyright 2000 by Joseph B. Marion, Information Pioneers Publ., South Woodstock, Connecticut. Paraphrasing/summarizing from page 40.

Northrup, Christiane, MD, *Women's Bodies, Womens' Wisdom*, Creating Physical and Emotional Health and Healing, copyright 1994 by Christiane Northrup, M. D., Bantam Books, a division of Bantam Doubleday Dell Publishing Group, Inc., New York, New York.

Rosenthal, M. Sara, foreword by Pratt, Suzanne G., M. D., F.A.C.O.G., *The Gynecological Sourcebook*, Third Edition, copyright 1994, 1995, 1997, 1999 by NTC/Contemporary Publishing Group, Lowell House, a division of NTC/Contemporary Publishing Group, Inc., Lincolnwood, Ill.

Sharon, Michael, *Complete Nutrition*, How to Live In Total Health, copyright 1989 by Michael Sharon, first published in the United Kingdom in 1989 by PRION, an imprint of Multimedia Books Limited, London, England.

The New Oxford Annotated Bible with The Apocrypha, New Revised Standard Version, edited by Bruce M. Metzger and Roland E. Murphy, copyright 1991, 1994 by Oxford University Press, Inc., New York, New York.

Treatment Option: Surgical Procedure, Stanford CVIR-Treatment Center, internet source pulled July 7, 2003, www.radiologicsurgery.com.

Uterine Fibroid Embolization Incision, Ad, *Ebony* magazine, 6/2002.

Walker, N. W., D.Sc., *Fresh Vegetable and Fruit Juices*, what's missing in your body?, copyright 1970 by Dr. Norman W. Walker, Published annually since 1936, formerly called Raw Vegetable Juices, revised and retitled Fresh Vegetable and Fruit Juices, 1978, Norwalk Press, Prescott, Arizona.

Wigmore, Ann, *The Wheatgrass Book*, copyright 1985 by Ann Wigmore and the Hippocrates Health Institute, Inc., published by Avery, a member of Penguin Putnam Inc.

Williams, Carmine E., M.D., *Excerpt from Dilation and Curettage*, internet source pulled July 7, 2003, www.emedicine.com, emedicine®, Instant Access to the Minds of Medicine.

References on menopause

Hall, Lynne L., Taking Charge of Menopause, *FDA Consumer*, Nov/Dec 99 Vol. 33, Issue 6, p17, 5p, 1c, 2bw.

Oliwenstein, Lori, That Certain Age, *Vegetarian Times*, 01648497, Jul99, Issue 263.

Shanahan, Kelly, M. D., Menopause: What is the Average Age?, Internet source: Family Health Resources, ivillagehealth.com, pulled 1/24/04.

Women's Health Weekly (NewsRx), September is National Menopause Awareness Month, 09/07/98, p11, 2/3p.

Internet sources (statistics)

Statistics reflected for U.S. women—uterine fibroid tumor activity. [Note: Worldwide activity/data would increase this epidemic significantly.] Sources: Women Magazine (www.jang.com.pk, Fibroid: causes, symptoms and treatment, May 2003, pulled 1/29/2004); National Institutes of Health— National Institute of Child Health and Human Development (www.nichd.nih.gov, Scientists On Step Closer to Cause of Uterine Fibroids, July 22, 2002, pulled 1/29/2004); the National Institute of Environmental Health Sciences (NIEHS) and the National Center for Research on Minority Health and Health Disparities (NCMHD) (www.niehs.nih.gov, Fibroid Growth Study, last modified Nov. 5, 2002, pulled 1/29/2004); University of Maryland Medicine (www.umm.edu, Uterine Fibroids, 2003, pulled 1/29/2004); the National Uterine Fibroids Foundation (www.nuff.org, Statistics [last update April 18, 2002], The Uterus [last update March 26, 2002], Uterine Fibroids [last update March 26, 2002], pulled 1/28/2004 1st two and 12/17/2003); Ebony magazine, Fibroid Tumors, March 2003, Vol. 58 Issue 5, p128, 1p, Johnson Publishing Company, pulled from Academic Search Premier Database, internet source 1/28/2004; Nutrition Health Review: The Consumer's Medical Journal, The Predicament of Choosing a Treatment for Uterine Fibroids, by Eleanor Mayfield, 1994 Issue 68, p12, 2p, pulled from EBSCO Host Research Database, Health Source, internet source 1/29/2004; The Medical Center online (www.mccg.org, Gynecological Health, Uterine Fibroids, MCCG is a registered trademark of The Medical Center of Central Georgia, pulled 12/17/2003); MayoClinic.com, Uterine Fibroids, by Mayo clinic staff, Feb. 25, 2002, pulled 12/17/2003 and; MEDLINEplus (www.nlm.nih.gov, link page, Uterine Fibroids, last page updated Dec. 15, 2003, pulled 12/17/2003).

Other Recommended Reading & Contacts

Rosemary Gladstar, *Herbal Healing for Women.*

Louise L. Hay, *You Can Heal Your Life.*

Jethro Kloss, *Back to Eden,* The Classic Guide to Herbal Medicine, Natural Foods and Home Remedies.

Dr. H. Emilie Cady, *Complete Works of H. Emilie Cady,* Lessons in Truth, How I Used Truth and God a Present Help.

Eldred B. Taylor, M. D., Board Certified Obstetrician/Gynecologist and author, *Are Your Hormones Making You Sick?,* Biblio distribution, available on Amazon.com. 1150 Hammond Dr., Building D, Suite 4230, Atlanta, GA 30328, (675) 205-4099.

HERS Foundation, Hysterectomy Educational Resources & Services. Provides information about alternatives to hysterectomies. www.hersfoundation.com

If I am not for myself, who will be for me? If I am not for others, who am I for? And if not now, when?

—Talmud—

Index

SPIRITUAL TREATMENTS

Change Your Thoughts,
Change Your Words

Change Your Words,
Change Your Actions

Change Your Actions,
Change Your World!

Affirmations

1 MY BODY IS WHOLE AND HEALTHY

2 EVERY CELL, ORGAN AND FIBER IN MY BODY IS WHOLE AND HEALTHY

3 ALL THINGS THAT GOD CREATED ARE EXPRESSIONS OF GOD (GOODNESS), I AM AN EXPRESSION OF GOD

4 GOD'S NATURAL LAW OF PERFECT HEALTH IS WORKING IN MY BODY

5 **MY BODY IS IN HARMONY**

6 FROM THE TOP OF MY HEAD ALL THE WAY DOWN THROUGH MY TOES I AM ENERGIZED

7 MY BODY GLOWS WITH HEALTH

Daily Thought

Sometimes when there is disharmony within the body it is time to pamper yourself from head to toe. Pamper your body with good, wholesome food, and a walk in the park on a beautiful sunny day, listening to children as they run and as they play. Pamper your mind by praying, relaxing and meditating. Pamper your life by being positive, upbeat and kind to all people. Most of all let God pamper you by your remembering that He is always here.

I am in total harmony. Every part of me functions precisely, divinely as it should. I pamper myself daily with wholesome food, exercise, prayer and good thoughts. I am aware of God's love for me and that He pampers me, too, by always being near. Thanks God. And So It Is!

"Pleasant words are like a honeycomb, sweetness to the soul and health to the bones." Proverbs 16:24

Affirmations

1 I AM AWARE OF THE GREAT POWER WITHIN ME

2 I LOVE AND ACCEPT MYSELF

3 WHEN I AM IN DOUBT, I GO WITHIN

4 I CAN DO ALL THINGS THROUGH CHRIST (THE SPIRIT OF ALL-KNOWING—DIVINE INTELLIGENCE, ALL-POWER) WHICH STRENGTHENS ME*

5 I AM ONE WITH ALL OF HUMANITY AND NATURE

6 **MY LIFE HAS MEANING**

7 THE CREATOR IS BLESSING ME WITH ITS PRESENCE

Daily Thought

Every life has meaning. Creation in itself is a beautiful and awesome thing. That means I am beautiful and awesome because I came out of Creation. The Creator must have a great imagination. I understand my connection with the Creator. I understand my life has meaning.

Each day as I face the world, I realize that in it I have meaning. Each day I actively participate in the world and share my smile, my kindness and my love. That's the meaning of my life. I am living it fully. Thanks God. And So It Is!

"Greater is He that is in you, than he that is in the world."
1 John 4:4

*Paraphrased from Philippians 4:13.

Affirmation

I AM EXERCISING MY FAITH MOMENT BY MOMENT

Daily Thought

Every day is an opportunity for me to exercise my faith. I am aware that it is God's good pleasure to give me the kingdom. The kingdom of good health, the kingdom of good thoughts, the kingdom of wonderful friendships, the kingdom of perfect work expressions, the kingdom of peace and the kingdom of love. I realize that by exercising my faith, I become fully aware of the spirit of God that is within me. And, as I recognize the spirit of God working within me, I am able to see the spirit of God all around me, and working through others, too. For this I am so grateful. As I exercise my faith by praying and being still, I know there is God, working out the perfect solution for me. Exercising my faith, my belief in the power of God, gives me the support I need. I know there is NO-THING too hard for God, so I release and I let God.

Today I decide to exercise my faith. I know that God is choosing the very best for me in all areas of my life, so I AM PATIENT. I exercise my faith by believing as though it is already done, because it is. All that concerns me is in divine order. Divine order is the highest order there is, and ever will be, and is the best possible outcome for me. I am exercising my faith moment by moment. I believe and I know that everything is all right. Thanks God. And So It Is!

"Now Faith is the substance of things hoped for, the evidence of things not yet seen." Hebrews 11:1

Affirmations

1 **I AM HAPPY**

2 I THINK AND SAY ONLY GOOD, HAPPY THINGS

3 I AM JOYFUL IN ALL I DO

4 HAPPINESS IS A STATE OF CONSCIOUSNESS, I **CHOOSE** TO BE HAPPY EVERY DAY

5 AS I GIVE OUT HAPPY THOUGHTS, I RECEIVE RESULTS THAT MAKE ME HAPPY

6 AS I THINK HAPPY THINGS, SO AM I

7 I THANK GOD FOR THE GIFT OF BEING HAPPY

Daily Thought

Happiness is a state of consciousness. It starts on the inside and moves outward. It requires a Smile, unlike sadness which requires a frown. As I focus on the things that bring me joy and peace and remove all the other stuff like confusion, doubt, fear and anxiety, I learn what happiness is all about. The Creator intends for me to be happy and provides the way for me. I keep my attention on God, which is all Goodness.

Each day I am happy because I know that happiness is a state of consciousness. **I choose to be happy**, and spread the love of God (all Goodness) to others. I know that God is always with me wanting the very best for me, this includes my being happy. Thanks God. And So It Is!

"Happy is the one that findeth wisdom, and getteth understanding." Proverbs 3:13

About The Author

Dr. Faye Hardaway, a *transpersonal/spiritual psychologist*, uplifts and teaches others through motivational speaking, workshops, seminars and writing.

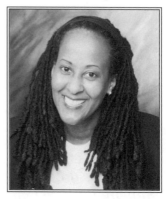

A *health enthusiast*, she has a passion for helping others from a *whole person* standpoint: *physical* (diet, nutrition and exercise), *mental* (thinking, the power of our thoughts and, subsequent actions), *feelings* (emotions) and *spiritual* (our connection with and knowledge of an unending reservoir of a majestic *creative power*, all-knowing *wisdom* and *strength* that is greater than anything we could possibly perceive at the personality/ego level).

Also holding a M.B.A. degree, concentrations in both Economics and Finance, Dr. Faye Hardaway has a *strong business background.* She has an interesting natural style of being able to blend spiritual attributes with the affairs of everyday living.

She is the author of the popular book *How to Get Your Boss to Work for You.*

Dr. Faye Hardaway is the founder of a *non-profit organization*, StepUp, Inc. This was her original planned project when she left a fifteen year corporate management career: to help those who have transitioned off the welfare system to not only find and maintain a job, but to become very successful as they increase their knowledge (*transcend—overcome any and all seemingly obstacles) in all major aspects of life.* Dr. Faye Hardaway is also a poet.

The Sun Began To Shine One Day

The sun began to shine one day and I saw the
wonders of the world so clear
I saw a less complicated path approaching near

I saw grass greener than ever before
I saw answers to long asked questions more and
more

I saw peace and happiness from a different view
I saw my attitude change to one fresh and new

I saw more friendly, warm and caring faces
I saw increased excitement in near and far places

I saw my value in life expanding each day
I saw a new set of words to express what I say

Yes, the sun began to shine one day and I saw It
and began to truly live!

Speaking, Workshops and Seminars

Dr. Faye Hardaway, Spiritual Psychologist, MBA, SC, is available for speaking, workshops and seminars.

Dr. Hardaway's seminars are highly interactive, using a whole person educational approach (creative and hands-on). Learning is to be Experienced!

Contact PositiveWay, Inc. for further information and bookings. PosWayInc@aol.com or (404) 691-5107.

Dr. Faye is on a mission:

To enlighten and inspire people through writing and speaking. She desires to see people overcome any and all seemingly challenges and to get on with living life more fully and joyously.

She truly believes that life is to be enjoyed and enthusiastically and wholeheartedly takes this message with her wherever she goes. She desires to touch each person she meets with a ray of sunshine.

The Creator and I are a Perfect Team

PositiveWay, Inc.

Where people go to be inspired

Quick Order Form

Please send me the following:

____*Fibroid Tumors Healed Naturally* $12.00

____*How To Get Your Boss To Work For You* $19.95

____*Spirituality In The Workplace* (Future Release)
price TBA

____Information on Other Future Releases

____Information on speaking/seminars

Company
name: _____

Name: _____

Address: _____

City:_____ State: _____Zip: _____

Telephone number: (___) _____

If making a purchase, please enclose a check or money order for the proper amount. Make payable to Positive Way, Inc. Send your payment with this order form to PositiveWay, Inc. P.O. Box, 310115 Atlanta, Georgia, 31131-0115.

_____# of Books ordering	$_____
plus Shipping and **Handling** **U.S.:** $4.00 for the first book shipped and $3.00 for each additional book **International:** $9.00 for the first book and $5.00 for each additional	$_____
Sales Tax (Georgia residents 7% metro Atlanta Fulton county, all others as applicable)	$_____
Total enclosed	$_____

PositiveWay, Inc.

Where people go to be inspired

Quick Order Form

Please send me the following:

____*Fibroid Tumors Healed Naturally* $12.00

____*How To Get Your Boss To Work For You* $19.95

____*Spirituality In The Workplace* (Future Release)
                                        price TBA

____Information on Other Future Releases

____Information on speaking/seminars

Company
name: _____

Name: _____

Address: _____

City:_____ State: _____Zip: _____

Telephone number: (____) _____

If making a purchase, please enclose a check or money order for the proper amount. Make payable to Positive Way, Inc. Send your payment with this order form to PositiveWay, Inc. P.O. Box, 310115 Atlanta, Georgia, 31131-0115.

____# of Books ordering $_____

plus Shipping and **Handling** $_____
U.S.: $4.00 for the first book shipped and
$3.00 for each additional book
International: $9.00 for the first book
and $5.00 for each additional

Sales Tax (Georgia residents 7% $_____
metro Atlanta Fulton county, all
others as applicable)

          Total enclosed $_____